HOME-VISITING STRATEGIES

Social Problems and Social Issues
Leon Ginsberg, Series Editor

Home-Visiting Strategies

A CASE-MANAGEMENT GUIDE
FOR CAREGIVERS

Terry Eisenberg Carrilio

THE UNIVERSITY OF SOUTH CAROLINA PRESS

Published by the University of South Carolina Press
Columbia, South Carolina 29208

www.sc.edu/uscpress

Manufactured in the United States of America

16 14 13 12 11 10 09 08 07   10 9 8 7 6 5 4 3 2 1

Library of Congress Cataloging-in-Publication Data

Carrilio, Terry Eisenberg.
  Home-visiting strategies : a case-management guide for caregivers / Terry Eisenberg Carrilio.
    p. cm. — (Social problems and social issues)
  Includes bibliographical references and index.
  ISBN-13: 978-1-57003-676-7 (pbk : alk. paper)
  ISBN-10: 1-57003-676-4 (pbk : alk. paper)
  1. Home-based family services—United States. 2. Family social work—United States. I. Title.
  HV699.C27 2007
  362.1'0425—dc22
                                                                    2006100533

Figure 4.3 was previously published as figure 1, "Sample Ecomap," in A. R. McPhatter (1991), Assessment revisted: A comprehensive approach to understanding family dynamics, *Families in Society* 72 (1): 15. Figure 4.4 was previously published as figure 1, "Culturagram," in E. P. Congress (1994), The use of culturagrams to assess and empower culturally diverse families, *Families in Society,* 75 (9): 532. Both figures are used by permission of Families in Society.

This book was printed on Glatfelter's Natures, a recycled paper with 50 percent post-consumer waste content.

This book is dedicated to my family, David, Sarah, Leah, and Brian,
for all of their patience and support and for reminding me that life goes on,
even when there is work to do, and to Eric, who paid attention

CONTENTS

ILLUSTRATIONS

SERIES EDITOR'S PREFACE

The tasks of human services workers in fields such as home health services, child welfare investigation and counseling, assistance to the elderly, community mental health, and work with people who have emotional and physical disabilities, often include visits to client homes.

Dr. Terry Carrilio, a long-time social work practitioner, educator, and researcher, provides those who practice social work and others who work in the human services with a guide to home visiting—how to prepare for, conduct, evaluate, and follow up with a visit.

It is a hallmark of human services work that the services we provide are personal and involve person-to-person contact. Although computers and data-processing software have been adapted to serving people, the personal, human touch always remains a central part of our work. And there is nothing quite as personal and dramatic in all the human services as the home visit.

This systematic, thorough, and sensitive book will be of assistance to all human service agencies and to those who are employed by them to reach and help clients who face all the social and personal problems with which such agencies deal. Most of the books in this series are about social issues and social facts. This book, *Home-Visiting Strategies: A Case-Management Guide for Caregivers,* is the first in the series to deal with the practice of human services—how to carry out a specific function. It is long overdue in the literature and provides help and guidance to employees who are assigned cases that require initial and, especially, continuing home visits in order to make the human services effort work.

We hope that this book will be only the first in a series of helpful publications designed to assist human services programs and workers in carrying out their challenging day-to-day jobs. The author knows the ins and outs of home visiting, but she also reassures readers about their own capacities for helping—helping them know the ways in which earlier knowledge may be applicable to new situations.

Of course, there are right and wrong ways to conduct home visits, and Dr. Carrilio takes note of both in this book as part of her guidance for those who conduct home visits—for family services, child welfare investigations, and all the other myriad tasks that are associated with home visiting, especially family support and carrying out the tasks of case management with clients.

This is a well-done guide by an experienced and ethical professional. We hope it will be useful and revealing for many readers for many years.

LEON GINSBERG

PREFACE

Over a period of several years I was fortunate enough to have had the opportunity to be involved in multiple family support home-visiting programs, and worked with policy makers, funders, administrators, and line staff in over twenty-five sites in California. These programs were primarily part of a series of initiatives by public and private funders in response to recent research findings about the importance of early childhood experiences and brain development, the impact of parental burden on family functioning, and the promise of early intervention and prevention programs. Having worked previously in programs providing community-based long term care for older adults and psychosocial rehabilitation with the severely and persistently mentally ill, it seemed to me that many of the principles of practice utilized in these two areas of practice could be transferred to work with vulnerable, overburdened families (Zeitz 1995). Work with these vulnerable groups reflects some commonalities:

1. Problems are multidimensional and layered.
2. The focal concerns do not lend themselves to a one-time quick fix but endure over time.
3. There is considerable risk lurking in the background.
4. The focus of interventions is often on "here-and-now" functioning.
5. The recipients of services may be reluctant and distrustful.
6. There is a strong commitment to empowerment.
7. The relationship between the helper and the client is an essential part of effective work.
8. There are often multiple helpers involved with a single client.

In the fields of aging and mental health services, case management is often conceptualized as the service that is being provided. Oftentimes these programs incorporate center-based group activities with in-home services. The client often has multiple service providers with a care manager coordinating and monitoring progress. In the world of family support, however, the discussion that I entered had to do with home visiting as a service. Initially I was puzzled, since home visiting is not actually a service, but is a description of the *location* of services. Plumbers provide services through home visits, as do fire and police. Some of us may even remember when the pediatrician provided medical care through home visits. When I entered the family support arena, I found a great deal of confusion and conflict about home-visiting models, and the effectiveness of home visiting. I must confess that from the beginning, I thought that we had confused the place that the service occurs with the service itself. As I examined many of the home-visiting program models (Martin 1999; Winter 1999; Olds

1999; Woods 1999; Culross 1999), it occurred to me that while it had not been articulated as such, many of these programs were, in fact, providing case-management services to families. Often direct services, such as direct developmental interventions with children and group-based parent education were included, but in all programs, home visitors were developing relationships, identifying strengths, enhancing coping and activities of daily-living skills, helping with problem solving, and coordinating resources. These activities are often included in definitions of case management. Because many overburdened families struggle with issues of transportation and time management the idea of providing home visits to engage families is imminently sensible. This is a strategy for delivering services. Early on I identified the home-visiting programs with which I was involved as family support case management being provided in the home.

Another feature that the family support programs had in common with the long-term case management programs for the elderly and the severely and persistently mentally ill was the use of multiple specialized providers. The case-management approach of coordinating several specialists and maintaining lines of communication is common in services for the elderly. In mental health, while the case-management model is used, it is often suggested that the specialists work together on teams. The ACT program (Stein and Santos 1998), in particular, articulates a model of team case management centered on the team's "ownership" of case responsibility. This approach reduces the dominance of any one paradigm when dealing with the kind of multilayered problems experienced by clients with mental illness. In looking at families coming in to family support programs, it appeared that many of these families were bringing parental developmental and mental health issues, substance abuse problems, health issues, parent-child relationship issues, economic, housing, educational, environmental, legal, relationship, cultural, and other dimensions into their current situations. It was obvious to me that one person could not possibly possess skills in all of these areas. These observations led to the development of a model of integrated team case management for working with overburdened families (Carrilio 2001).

The integrated team case-management approach allows multiple specialists to work with a family in a collaborative manner. It also permits for an integration of home-based and center-based services. The approach borrows heavily from principles of psychosocial rehabilitation. Family support teams are challenging not only because the differential training of members leads to different paradigms of service, but also because it contains individuals at different levels of education. Clearly, a good team leader must be highly skilled in group process and be able to manage the tension between needing to work with families in a collaborative manner and each team member's desire to do it their way.

During much of the 1990s and the early 2000s what I have called the "model wars" raged on, diverting attention prematurely to the effectiveness of programs when we were not yet able to even articulate exactly what the programs were. There is important research about intervention and prevention programs with vulnerable families, some of which will be discussed in chapter 1 and elsewhere in the book. However, I have always felt that we jumped too quickly to prove effectiveness and had barely articulated the programs. In fact, home-visiting programs differ considerably with respect to staffing, how and when families are recruited, duration of services, array of services, intensity of services, and expected outcomes. In order to know if we are being effective, it would seem important to be really clear about what we are trying to accomplish. It is important to integrate policy, research, and practice in program logic models and to explicitly connect these logic models to program implementation and quality management planning. Once we can convince ourselves that there is a sound program model that has been well implemented, then we are in a position to evaluate what we have done and how well we have done it.

As I became more involved in program development and evaluation in family support it was difficult to find training information for the teams. I had the opportunity, with the help of the California Department of Social Services and the Stuart Foundation to develop and provide a forty-hour training program to hundreds of home visitors from 1997 to 2002. This training was developed with colleagues, and relied heavily on several working position papers, along with ongoing literature reviews. While we found many articles about which models of home visiting were more effective, there was not very much available about how to actually DO family support home visiting. We developed training manuals specifically for the training, and these ended up being disseminated to programs in many states. I kept waiting for a how-to book that I could give to supervisors, administrators, and home visitors to help them with their work. In 2003 I prepared a detailed how-to guide, *A Step by Step Guide to Home Visiting* that partially addressed this need.

With the current book I hope to offer the reader some of what I have learned in the development, operation, and evaluation of family support programs. It is intended for administrators, supervisors, and, most important, the home visitors themselves. I hope that it provides some focused hands-on information that is useful in working with vulnerable families.

I have organized the book so that it starts with an overview of home visiting and case management and then moves on to discuss, in some detail, the steps of the case-management process carried out by the home visitor. Chapters 1 and 2 will be of most interest to program administrators and supervisors, as these chapters address issues of theory, research, and organizational context. In chapter 1 some of the underlying conceptual frameworks of family support home visiting are explored. Chapter 2 explores the ways in which the organization and program structure influence the home visitor's activities. Chapters 3 through 7 are specifically intended as a hands-on guide for home visitors. Chapter 3 explores the initial stages of engaging families in family support home-visiting services. Chapters 4 through 7 present the key steps of case management involved in providing home-visiting services. Chapter 8 directs attention to some of the issues surrounding work in teams, and should be of interest to home visitors and to program administrators and supervisors. Chapters 8 and 9 will be of interest to program administrators and supervisors. Chapter 10 introduces some ways in which home-visiting and office-based activities can be integrated. Also, program administrators and supervisors will find some hands-on advice for setting up documentation systems and managing quality and data collection in chapter 10. In order to offer a sense of how to work with the concepts presented in chapters 3 through 7, the reader will be introduced to the Rodriguez family and will follow their trajectory through a home-visiting program.

ACKNOWLEDGMENTS

I wrote this book with the support of colleagues, students, and staff with whom I have worked over the years. I want to thank David Chadwick and Geri Beattie for believing in me and for giving me the space to develop family support programs and try out new concepts. The staff members of the Family Support Programs at the Chadwick Center (formerly the Center for Child Protection) at Children's Hospital–San Diego were supportive and flexible. Their willingness to follow new paths led to some truly amazing programs. The original South Bay Home Support team, including Christine Pemberton, Elsa Rodriguez, Sofia Bordson, Joan Dicciani, and Ruth Buccio, patiently worked with me to clarify and make real many of the practice ideas contained in this book. Subsequent South Bay Home Support teams, as well as the Healthy Families–San Diego teams made it possible to develop and understand many of the concepts that have found their way into this book.

Marge Kelley, Eloise Anderson, and Eileen Carroll provided early funding and policy support for the development of the programs that this book is based upon. John Landsverk provided important ballast as the family support home-visiting ship raced through uncharted waters. His insistence on using strong evidence and on viewing every component critically served to strengthen the conceptual base and enhanced program operations.

Thanks go as well to the Social Policy Institute staff, who worked diligently to refine the concepts of integrated team case management and maintained a strong focus on quality management. Special thanks go to Malia Adler, Beth Sheffield, and Lara Gamble for their diligence in implementing and troubleshooting the management information system that became an integral part of quality management and program operations.

Many of the concepts underlying the family support home-visiting concepts presented in this book were refined with the help of Mary Clare Heffron, Donna Weston, and Deborah Bremmond. It was a pleasure working with them on early efforts to train home visitors and disseminate a best practices family support home-visiting model.

Leon Ginsberg provided support and guidance in moving the book from a concept to a reality. Many thanks go to him for this.

My final thanks go to all of the home visitors who attended our Cal–SAHF and ABC trainings, as well as to my students at San Diego State University School of Social Work. Their questions and efforts to apply ideas "on the ground" have helped to anchor the principles and practices suggested in this book.

HOME-VISITING STRATEGIES

ONE

Home Visiting

A FAMILY-SUPPORT STRATEGY

The future of any society depends in great part on the ability of each generation to transmit values, knowledge, and skills to the next generation and to provide the support, security, and continuity that is needed for the new generation to develop the capacity for autonomy. In developed Western societies, families are responsible for providing an early environment that will prepare children to engage as citizens in the larger society. Conventional wisdom tells us that a child who feels loved and secure and who has had "good enough" parenting (Winnicott 1965) will arrive at school ready to learn and to embark on an educational journey to develop the necessary social skills to function in his/her society. While industrialized Western societies differ in the amount of financial, in-kind, and social supports offered to the family, it is clear from the plethora of "smart baby" books and parenting guides that both parents and society assume that the burden of preparing a child who is ready to function with his/her peers rests with the child's family.

The infant and young child embedded in a "good enough" family develops the cognitive, emotional, motor, moral, and social skills that enable him/her to begin the long process of socialization required in order to achieve adult standing in a complex social context. Although current Western societies possess their share of critics, most children follow a developmental path that results in their graduation to full, functional adulthood. In most cases this involves, at some level, the achievement of a stable sense of self, reasonably good self-esteem, vocational skills, social skills, the capacity for stable, long-term relationships, and the capacity to negotiate institutions and social systems effectively. Yet, there are some families and children who, for a variety of reasons, are not able to achieve the basic level of adult functioning required to thrive in their social context.

These families are often considered socially excluded (Buchanan et al. 2004) because they are having difficulty providing for their members on one or several dimensions. The concept of social exclusion draws a strong connection between poverty and the exclusion of some members of society from the benefits of the wider society (Buchanan et al. 2004; Katz and Pinkerton 2003). In a recent report on social policies to reduce the risk of social exclusion, Buchanan points out that social exclusion is multidimensional and includes poverty, housing, and environmental deficits, inadequate early education and childcare, lack of access to education and poor academic achievement, poor health, and vulnerable families whose children often require child protection (Buchanan et al. 2004). These are families who are overburdened, in that they are vulnerable to social exclusion. If we view families from an ecological point of view, that is, considering the interaction of family characteristics with characteristics in the larger social and physical context, the concept of being overburdened can be understood as representing an imbalance between the demands placed upon the family and the resources it has available to manage these demands. This leads to increased vulnerability for all family members. In this light vulnerability is not a fixed state, but a dynamic balance between the individual and family's capacities and resources and the burdens and challenges that they confront at any given time (Davies 1999).

We all experience vulnerability differently, and much depends on the dynamics of a particular moment. For instance most of us would experience a flat tire while driving as an annoyance; however, if we were to experience that flat tire on the way to a job interview, depending on how late we were, how much we wanted the job, and other factors, including our general emotional status *that day,* the flat tire could easily precipitate an anxiety state. The point here is that an external stressor, the flat tire, is real and would be acknowledged by all to be annoying; however, the level of stress experienced would depend heavily on the circumstances of the moment. Daily events may become overwhelming because of accumulated stress and overloading of an individual's capacities to problem solve and manage the tensions created by events.

For a variety of reasons, both personal, and external to the family system, the overburdened family often finds itself in an overextended, hyperanxious state in which it becomes difficult to function effectively. The overburdened family often experiences multiple, frequently co-occurring, difficulties with relationships, events, and institutions. The accumulation of pressure may result in a state of helplessness in which individual family members feel unable to do anything to resolve the stresses they are experiencing. There are many reasons that a family might be experiencing overwhelming stress. Sometimes the stresses are contextual, such as living in a violent neighborhood, living in poverty, being a single parent, experiencing unemployment, or living in substandard housing. Factors related to the individual's development and current internal state might also influence the experience of stress. For instance, being under the influence of drugs or alcohol, or experiencing withdrawal from these substances, unresolved or unmanaged mental health issues, and the parent's own history of abuse or developmental trauma (Kernberg 1994; Van der Kolk and Fisler 1994; Van der Kolk et al. 1994) may affect the capacities of family members to cope with even minor problems in daily living. Additional stress can be placed upon a family if there are children closely spaced in age, children with learning or behavioral problems, criminal activity, or unresolved relationship issues both within and outside of the family. Families who are vulnerable and socially excluded may be hard to reach (Mori 2005), and programs that aim simply to address the more concrete components of the problem, such as poverty, housing, or education may miss the powerful, sometimes multigenerational psychological impact of social exclusion upon families (Buchanan et al. 2004).

Family-support programs are intended to help vulnerable families move beyond learned helplessness and to develop a sense of efficacy and competence.

Over the past twenty years the concept of providing support to families in order to increase resiliency and reduce vulnerability has been an important part of the child welfare and child development literature. There is increasing evidence that prevention and broad-based support for families do lead to positive results (Karoly et al. 1998; Sweet and Appelbaum 2004; Buchanan et al. 2004; Hahn et al. 2005). Unfortunately much of the research in the area of family support is difficult to interpret and specific program characteristics leading to the development of effective interventions do not emerge consistently from the studies (Sweet and Appelbaum 2004; Chaffin, Bonner and Hill 2001; Gomby 1999; Culross 1999). We will return to this later in the chapter, but at present, it is important to first understand more about family-support programs and how they are intended to help vulnerable families.

FAMILY-SUPPORT PROGRAMS

Family-support programs are intended to increase resiliency by reducing vulnerability factors and increasing protective factors for children and families. An effective family-support program will 1) intervene to reduce the vulnerability factors and increase the protective factors in the family and its individual members, and 2) address community and environmental vulnerabilities and protective factors. Family-support programs cannot operate in isolation; there must be administrative and financial support as well as a connection to the community being served. Many family-support programs focus on issues of prevention, early childhood interventions, and parental capacity building with the intention of improving overall family resiliency.

Complex, multilevel, multifocused interventions meeting the family's unique needs are often required. There has been a great deal of debate about the effectiveness of early-childhood prevention programs. Much of the debate centers on what types of programs are most effective, how long it takes to realize results, and what results are realistic. Research continues to demonstrate the importance of the early years in social and cognitive development (Shonkoff and Phillips 2000). The long-lasting negative effects of trauma and disorganization in family life are also receiving support in the literature (Buka and Earls 1993; Fonagy 1998; Illig 1998; Kernberg 1994; Kotulak 1995; Van der Kolk and Fisler 1994; Anda et al. 2002; Dube et al. 2003).

The literature on child development, trauma, and adult psychopathology supports the notion that protective factors developed in the first few years, particularly the first three years of life, can serve the individual well in the face of later stresses and strains (Rutter 1987; Applegate and Bonnovitz 1995a; Van der Kolk et al. 1994; Carrilio and Walter 1984; Emde 1996; Kotulak 1995; Kernberg 1994). Rutter has clarified the importance of seeing resilience as a process, with the balance of protective and vulnerability factors changing as a result of intrapersonal or extrapersonal environmental stresses (Rutter 1987).

SIDEBAR 1.1

Factors Associated with Social Exclusion and Vulnerability

- History of abuse/neglect—may be multigenerational
- History of violence in the home
- History of substance abuse—may be multigenerational
- Limited parenting skills
- Unrealistic expectations of self and others
- Economic instability and insufficiency
- Isolation
- Few resources or supports
- Limited problem-solving skills
- Disempowered/disconnected from community
- Limited communications skills
- One or more family members with health, learning, mental health, and/or behavior problems
- Mental illness of the parent or child
- Difficulties managing activities of daily life
- Poverty, unemployment, or underemployment
- Low educational achievement

Families and individuals who are over-burdened and overwhelmed by the presence of vulnerability factors may easily demonstrate classic signs of learned helplessness (Seligman 1975). This construct becomes important in identifying and working with overburdened families, because frequently the negative consequences of learned helplessness and an external locus of control are the "symptoms" which call a family to the attention of social-service providers. The relationships between child abuse and neglect and parental depression and mental health problems are established in the literature. The family we define as overburdened is one for whom the challenges and vulnerabilities they experience outweigh the protective factors. The challenges faced by these families include 1) parental developmental and identity issues, 2) difficulties with the activities of daily living, 3) disturbances in the parent/child relationship, and 4) multiple problems or risk factors and involvement with multiple, sometimes contradictory, systems.

These challenges often result from the parent's own experiences in growing up. The parent develops characteristic internalized emotional patterns and expectations as a result of his/her own experiences. These internalized expectations influence the parent's ability to regulate self-esteem and to engage in holding and mirroring activities with the child. Mirroring and holding activities refer to the way in which the parent and child engage each other in a mutual interaction; these terms are often applied in observations of parent/child attachment behaviors. The parent's own developmental difficulties can affect his/her ability to coordinate expectations about the child with developmental realities and with the temperamental and constitutional realities presented by the child (Emde 1996; Applegate and Bonnovitz 1995b; Pipp-Siegel and Pressman 1996). The parent's own experiences also have a tremendous impact upon his/her ability to problem solve, make responsible judgments, control impulsive behaviors, and engage in help seeking behavior.

Overburdened families often have difficulty accessing existing community resources. Sometimes minor barriers or misunderstandings result in the family not accessing needed services. Sometimes they become familiar with one provider and try to use that provider for everything. They often have difficulty articulating their needs in a way in which helping organizations can respond to them effectively, and they frequently jump from one crisis to the next in an attempt to get help for themselves.

Many vulnerable families struggle with day-to-day concrete issues, such as housing and basic necessities. Abraham Maslow's (Maslow 1954) concept of a hierarchy of needs is particularly useful in working with families whose day-to-day lives often appear chaotic and crisis ridden. Maslow suggests that the basic needs of hunger, affection, and security take precedence over higher needs such as self-actualization, altruism, and philosophical searches for value and justice. The concrete needs of day-to-day life are very real for these families, and must be addressed before they are able to engage in self-reflection, struggle with past issues, and learn new coping skills.

A common mistake made with many overburdened families is that of pushing them toward psychological growth while they are still experiencing anxiety and uncertainty in basic areas of life, such as food, shelter, and security. Many of these families are struggling with poverty and limited personal and community resources. While having a social-work case manager cannot resolve all of these problems, participating in a family-support program *can* help the family to work with their limited resources and to make best use of additional community resources. For many families the anxieties of resolving day-to-day issues are reduced through linkages with community resources and the new skills they develop as they participate in the program.

Family-support home visiting represents a service *philosophy* consisting of several component services, usually organized around *home visiting* as a core service strategy for the purpose of improving family

---

SIDEBAR 1.2

Examples of Challenges Faced by Overburdened, Vulnerable Families

Parental development and identity
- Immature or disturbed internalized emotional patterns
- Difficulties with self-esteem regulation
- Underdeveloped capacity for concern
- Difficulties with mirroring and holding

Difficulties with activities of daily living (ADL)
- Immature or problematic problem-solving skills
- Immature or inappropriate judgment
- Reactive, difficulty planning
- Use of violence to express needs and feelings
- Difficulty accessing and using resources
- Difficulty identifying and meeting needs of family members
- Financial disarray
- Criminal involvement
- Difficulty maintaining adequate housing, income
- Health concerns not sufficiently addressed
- Struggle with time management and meeting expectations

Disturbances in family relationships
- Passive—not in charge, or conversely, overcontrolling
- Inconsistent, unstructured expectations
- Misunderstanding or lack of knowledge of normal development
- Attachment problems
- Difficulties with intimacy
- Violence and abuse

Multisystem concerns
- Criminal justice
- Child welfare
- Income maintenance/social welfare
- Educational system
- Housing
- Transportation
- Health
- Childcare

self-sufficiency (Kagan, Powell, Weisbourd, and Zigler 1987; Kagan and Neville 1993; Goetz and Peck 1994; Carrilio 1998). Families receive individualized help in their own homes and are provided with a safe environment to practice new skills and learn to utilize resources available to them in the community. They are also given opportunities to engage in center-based programs that address the social and cognitive skill development needs of both parents and children. Family-support home visiting is an effective service delivery *strategy* for programs attempting to prevent, reduce, and treat adverse health, social, and economic outcomes (Howe et al. 1999; Klass 1996; Karoly et al. 1998). Family-support home visiting represents a range of interventions aimed at supporting families to prevent and ameliorate the significant difficulties they experience. Programs differ with respect to staffing levels, funding, duration, and intensity. The best programs integrate research findings into policy and program development, and insist that the program structure and process of program delivery reflect the conceptual foundations of the program.

Even the most apparently impaired individuals and families possess strengths and qualities that can be built upon. Family-support home-visiting programs emphasize strengths, pragmatism, and social adaptation. Vulnerable families, for complex reasons related to personal history, resources, and parenting skills, may at times place one or more family members at risk, resulting in the intervention of social control agents such as the police, mental health agencies, or child protective services. A focus on strengths and on enhancing community functioning is implemented within a context of maintaining safety and well-being for all family members. A key goal is that of enabling individuals and families identified as overburdened or dysfunctional to develop and maintain the skills and coping strategies necessary to function independently in the community. Some of the families served in family-support programs may be involuntary, and some families will have already been identified as high risk. Yet it is possible to approach the helping relationship from a strengths-based perspective that embraces a philosophy of acceptance, empowerment, and normalcy, and avoids preoccupation with dysfunction and pathology. This is not to say that the shortcomings of the family or its members are ignored, but simply that problems are less at the center of attention than are those aspects of the family that reflect health, strength, and normality.

Strengths-based program structures tend to be empowering and egalitarian, with an emphasis on involving the family members as much as possible. A strengths-based family-support program seeks to provide experiential social learning opportunities by breaking down everyday activities into small parts, each of which can be mastered and integrated by the family members. There is a focus on solving here-and-now problems, resolving difficulties with material resources such as food, shelter, and medical care, reducing dependent behavior, increasing coping skills, and developing community resources for families. The goal is not to "cure" dysfunction, but rather the acquisition and maintenance of the basic skills needed to survive and thrive independently in the community.

Family members are seen as partners in the process, and there is a great deal of attention paid to issues of wellness and taking responsibility for one's own goals. The tone is upbeat and the focus of interventions is on the tangible, here-and-now issues of everyday life. Family members are encouraged to remain involved and to engage actively in social learning and resocialization activities. Family-support home-visiting programs deal with the family member in his/her current situation and attempts to work with both the environment and the family member to reach goals and maintain functioning. There is also recognition that even the most concrete, mundane event has learning and therapeutic potential. This requires recognizing what the family member's actual skills are, rather than what they are hoped to be. It also involves recognizing that learning a skill in one setting or functioning adequately in one environment does not guarantee that as the family member moves into a new situation these skills will be used successfully.

Often home visiting is considered as a strategy when it is difficult for people to get to the office. It is also a way to work around issues of transportation and time management, especially in the early stages of the relationship with a helping professional. One way to think about home visiting is that it is a strategy to assist with engaging families who might otherwise fall through the cracks. Essentially home visiting brings the services to the family. Especially with reluctant or disorganized families, home visiting is a way of meeting the client where the client is. Later I will look at the importance of knowing when the family has engaged and delineating the fine line between facilitating service delivery and acceptance and colluding with behavior patterns that may be self-defeating.

In keeping with the social context in which we work, social work, nursing, teaching, and even some elements of law enforcement in the United States have struggled since their earliest development with the balance between supporting and sanctioning troubled families (Hancock and Pelton 1989). It is a truism for most professionals that simply providing services without a strategy, plan, or focus may not be useful and may even do harm. It is also well recognized that in a democracy, individuals cannot be forced to comply with services, and in fact, have the right to refuse those services in many instances. On the other hand, there is a concern that the unmet needs of at-risk families and individuals will result in expensive problems in health, criminal justice, and lost wages in the future. These questions are often related to considerations of the nature of voluntary services and the extent to which public and private organizations can exert coercion in the service of changing families.

Programs referred to as "family-support" programs cover a wide range of services and target populations and occur in a variety of settings. These programs differ along a number of dimensions that together define the structure, integration, and philosophy of family support. There is a tendency to use family support both as a method of prevention and a method of intervention. Program goals and the specific goals of the program may dictate significant differences in the skills and education home visitors will require. Likewise, depending upon the underlying conceptual model, programs

■

SIDEBAR 1.3

Useful Web Sites

- Adverse Childhood Experiences Study: http://www.acestudy.org/aboutus.php
- Family Support America: http://www.familysupportamerica.org/content/home.htm
- Healthy Families America: http://www.healthyfamiliesamerica.org/home/index.shtml
- Harvard Family Research Project (HFRP): http://www.gse.harvard.edu/hfrp/projects/ost_participation.html
- Home Instruction Program for Parents of Preschool Youngsters (HIPPY): http://www.hippyusa.org/
- National Center for Children in Poverty: http://www.nccp.org/
- Parents as Teachers: http://www.parentsasteachers.org/

will offer differing intensities of services and for differing amounts of time. We need to move beyond simply cataloging programs (Culross 1999; Martin 1999, Winter 1999; Olds 1999; Woods 1999) and look toward what systems and principles will accomplish which ends. Systems, by definition, involve multiple levels of attention, including the community, the economy, and the larger social-political context. A system of family support provides services 1) *in vitro* (that is, in locations conducive to the family's needs, such as home, family resource centers, and other locations in the community), 2) through intensive team case management, and 3) to children and parents identified as overburdened.

Family support as a concept contains some dilemmas. Should we focus our attention on the supportive aspects of improving family functioning and well-being, or should our attention be focused upon the inherent social control aspects of improving behavior in the community (Hancock and Pelton 1989)? In reality, these dialectical relationships do not lend themselves to simple resolution on one side or another. For example, one can view the development of impulse control as both a supportive function which enhances efficacy, competence, and enables the child to operate successfully in school and social settings; at the same time we can see that the community's interest in this outcome may be a result of concern over the negative health, social, and legal consequences associated with poor impulse control. Most professionals engaged in family-support work struggle with this dialectic in the area of voluntary versus required services. Again, a part of our purpose may well be to engage a family in activities that we see as valuable to enhancing their ability to thrive interpersonally, and in the community. Yet, we struggle with the dilemmas of what to do if the family does not agree or show interest in our offer of support.

The questions of how much freedom a family has to refuse support are complex and often vex professionals in the field. In thinking through our responses, we learn that underlying values and social context may have a tremendous impact upon the way we perform outreach and how we choose to engage families in services. Ultimately any family-support system will need to answer questions about what purpose services are to provide, which outcomes are desirable, and which are undesirable. Additionally key decisions need to be made with respect to the role of the client family and the professional in the system.

In the 1998 Rand report, *Investing in Our Children: What We Know and Don't Know about the Costs and Benefits of Early Childhood Interventions*, Karoly and her coauthors, along with other reviewers, have concluded that well-thought-out, well-implemented programs of family support offered early in a child's life can very well lead to the reduction of vulnerability and the enhancement of positive outcomes later in the child's life. A recent review of evaluations of home-visiting interventions, published by the David and Lucille Packard Foundation, finds that the data on many of these programs is equivocal and that there is a wide variability in programs and results. The recommendations in this report include a recognition that expectations for a single service intervention need to be modest, particularly when the complexity of the problems facing overburdened families is considered. Additionally the report recommends that quality management systems be implemented in home-visiting programs and that model fidelity and implementation issues be seriously considered.

Many family-support programs, based on theory, practice, professional codes of ethics, and preference, also share some key underlying values and assumptions about the role of the family and of the helper. Many home-visiting programs are intended to work with individuals and families suffering from serious disorganization and dysfunction in carrying out the tasks of day-to-day living. This is an intensely and minutely practical approach which focuses heavily on teaching the practical skills needed to function independently in the community. While insight and traditional psychotherapeutic approaches may be part of an overall service plan, there is a recognition that skill development and functioning in everyday life are necessary in order to effectively utilize more traditional insight-oriented interventions.

Evaluations of these programs have often been high-stakes propositions (Sweet and Appelbaum 2004; Sherwood 2005; Hahn et al. 2005), with policy, funding, and program structure hanging in the balance. The gold standard of randomized clinical studies was established early on, and although there are researchers suggesting alternative research paradigms (Daro 2005; Hahn et al. 2005), home-visiting programs continue to be reviewed in a high-pressure environment with high expectations. The proverbial silver bullet—the intervention or combination of interventions that will improve family functioning and reduce adverse outcomes has yet to be identified. The findings emerging from evaluations of home-visiting programs are conflicting and difficult to interpret (Chaffin, Bonner, and Hill 2001; Daro and Cohn-Donnelly 2002a; Sweet and Appelbaum 2004; Duggan et al. 2004; Hahn et al. 2005).

HOME-VISITING AND FAMILY-SUPPORT PROGRAMS

We often consider family-support, home-visiting, and early-intervention programs as identical, perhaps because interventions with these names often share similar or related goals, theories, and intervention strategies. Frequent goals of these programs include

1. Supporting optimal family functioning
2. Achieving positive health and developmental outcomes for all family members
3. Improving educational and occupational opportunities
4. Improving children's cognitive development and school readiness
5. Preventing or reducing adverse outcomes
6. Strengthening and supporting families and communities

These goals are efforts to reduce the high social costs associated with such inter-laced adverse outcomes as low intellectual functioning, underemployment, family violence, child abuse and neglect, delinquency, adult criminality, substance abuse, and poor health. An underlying assumption has been that improved cognitive, emotional, and social functioning by family members will reduce the incidence and effects of adverse circumstances and generally enhance individual and community well-being. Common theoretical foundations include efficacy theory, ecological theory, attachment theory, object relations theory, psychosocial rehabilitation theory, and assertive case management. Less common, but potentially offering important contributions, are theories of cognitive functioning and moral development. The different approaches that are identified with home visiting are often the result of the way that program developers and administrators address theoretical orientations, community and policy contexts, and funding support. In the following section, we will talk a little about some of the theories that underlie programs that use home visiting as an intervention. These theories are not mutually exclusive and are often combined in a single program. Recent work has focused on the interaction of the child, the parent, and the community to promote or inhibit resiliency (Shonkoff and Phillips 2000; Davies 1999; Howe et al. 1999). Although there are overlapping theoretical frameworks and values assumptions, home-visiting programs differ along several key dimensions, as illustrated in sidebar 1.4.

SIDEBAR 1.4

Services That Are Referred to as "Home-Visiting Programs" Differ in Many Ways

- Who does the home visiting?
  - Professionals
  - Agents of social control (police, child protective workers)
  - Paraprofessionals
  - Volunteers
- Whether the home visiting is voluntary or mandated
- Duration of visits—range from one contact to several years
- Intensity of visits—from several times a week to quarterly or less frequent visits
- Service mix—from home visits only to comprehensive center-based services for children and parents
- Point of contact—can range from prenatal, preventive contact to contact during or after a crisis (police intervention, hospitalization, child protective intervention, and so on)
- Purpose of the home visit—this can range from support, to education, to counseling, to home health provision, to surveillance and investigation

It is important to remember that home visiting is not a service in and of itself. It is a strategy that enables the provider to perform a service. People with different backgrounds do home visits—nurses, social workers, police officers, probation officers, teachers, occupational therapists, counselors, physical therapists, volunteers, and community workers frequently provide some in-home services. Individuals providing in-home services may range from community volunteers to licensed professionals in several fields. Providers range from police officers, to nurses, to social workers to indigenous community paraprofessionals, and they carry out a multitude of programmatic goals. Most of us are familiar with home visits by the plumber, electrician, exterminator, and other providers of household services. In these cases, the home visit is the locus of a specific service, provided by a trained person, such as fixing a leaky faucet, installing an electrical fixture, or ridding the house of ants. The example should make it clear that the family-support home visitor, like other home visitors, should be trained and should be entering the home with a clear purpose.

The task of a family-support home visitor will be to intensively build skills in the home and then assist parents and children to practice and integrate these skills in a variety of situations over a period of time. The overburdened family is extremely vulnerable and requires substantial support in order to simply carry on everyday activities. Family-support home visiting has at its foundation a concept of development and learning that suggests that before a family member can risk change or growth, he or she must develop a sense of being in a secure, cohesive context. To ask an overburdened parent or difficult child to change behavior, or to insist upon autonomy without first assuring some continuity or stability upon which they can rely, is to invite increased disorganization and deterioration in functioning. For this reason the home visitor attends to structure and consistency, enabling family members to count on continuity, and to experience, in a supportive environment, the consequences (both positive and negative) of their own actions. There is a recognition that the family requires a comprehensive and coordinated service array in order to both learn and apply the skills needed to function independently in the community. In a later chapter we will explore the ways in which home-based and center-based services can work together to help families accomplish this integration.

CASE-MANAGEMENT AND FAMILY-SUPPORT HOME VISITING

Case management, in the context of family-support home visiting, represents the activities of the home visitor and the team which assist the family in resolving day-to-day logistical problems, negotiating systems, and linking activities to the service plan. Ongoing problem-solving case coordination responsibilities range from brokering resources to advocating for the family as it negotiates the many systems with which it is involved, to providing direct counseling and psychoeducational interventions. Many of the concepts used in psychosocial rehabilitation and principles of clinical case management from the field of mental health (Zeitz 1995) are useful in working with vulnerable families. Some family-support advocates might fear that this pathologizes the family. Yet, there is a high incidence of clinical depression, substance abuse, and consequent sense of helplessness among families identified as vulnerable, socially excluded, or overburdened (Carrilio 2006; Landsverk et al.2001). This may lead to a functional status and a need for ongoing case management support similar to what one sees in mental health populations.

The home visitor works with the family to identify effective strategies for linking with community resources and for meeting their personal goals. For many overburdened families, the combination of past experience, lack of skills in negotiating systems, and personal dynamics often lead to self-defeating and frustrating interactions with the organizations and institutions with which they interact. The home visitor may actually go to the school or the unemployment office with the parents, and assist them with planning the contact, anticipatory problem solving, clarifying the goals of the contact, and modeling ways to communicate in ways which are effective within these often complex systems.

The home visitor works with the family to develop decision trees and crisis plans so that the family has already practiced using resources appropriately *before* a crisis. The home visitor helps the family to identify and utilize its strengths and resources, and to identify a stepwise approach to problem solving so that family members do not become overwhelmed. As an example, a mother who typically uses the hospital emergency room when her child develops a high fever might be helped to develop a checklist of symptoms, a telephone list of people to call with questions, and be helped to develop a relationship with a primary care health provider with whom she can make an appointment. By helping the mother to identify the symptoms and teaching her to gather information from the nurse, the home visitor, or the primary care practitioner, the home visitor helps the parent to get care for the child sooner and more appropriately. Successfully managing these day-to-day crises is an empowering experience for families, and over time the home visitor will teach the family to develop problem solving and coping skills so that the family can more effectively provide its own problem-solving case coordination.

Case management is a core organizing principle for family-support programs. The case management approach should be focused on an individualized family service plan, which is regularly reviewed and monitored. No single service strategy is a stand-alone intervention. Services are embedded within a comprehensive and integrated service matrix, which is bound together through the case management.

Case management involves more than simple linking, brokering, or referring to other services. The case management function serves as the connecting process among the services utilized both within the team and from outside resources. It is makes a "holding environment" operational (Winnicott 1965; Applegate and Bonnovitz 1995a) and includes more than instrumental activities because it is dependent upon the development of a relationship between the team and the family. Case management should be viewed as a clinical intervention that requires the input of the entire team. It is therapeutic but does not always involve therapy.

The case management function is family focused. While this means many things, one of the very concrete, structural considerations includes flexible hours so that staff is working when clients are available.

In practice, this means that home visits may occur evenings, weekends, or at the workplace, and center-based activities should be scheduled to meet evening and weekend schedules as well. An additional benefit to scheduling the program to meet the needs of the families is that it is more likely that fathers/significant others will participate under these circumstances.

STRUCTURING FAMILY-SUPPORT PROGRAMS

Most of the debates about home-visiting and family-support models center around structural aspects of the models. For example, debate continues about the use of resources for primary prevention in the face of the tremendous needs of tertiary care populations. There is debate about who prevention services should target. Should services be targeted or universal? Are these early childhood programs best with high-risk or low-risk families? Is a program that has been shown to be effective with primary prevention equally effective as a secondary prevention approach? Other questions often argued include:

1. How long and how intensive should services be?
2. What services should actually be provided?
3. Should services target the parent, child, or both?
4. Should services be home based, center based, or both?
5. What are we trying to achieve with early intervention services?
6. What type of staff should be providing the intervention services?

As reviews of existing studies and programs have indicated, different goals, different measures, and different interventions abound.

In a recent review of case management practices in mental health services, Rapp and Goscha (2004) identified ten characteristics of effective case management programs:

1. The service is delivered as much as possible by the case manager directly, with less focus on the use of multiple brokered services.
2. Natural supports and resources in the community, such as family members, friends, and employers are seen as partners.
3. Services are delivered in the community, with a great deal of outreach and contact in vivo.
4. Case management is carried out in teams, with either full team case management or individual case management under the supervision of a highly trained professional.
5. Responsibility for services is with the case manager, rather than with a system of care.

6. Case managers may range in skill and training, from indigenous workers to highly trained professionals. It is necessary for the case manager to receive supervision from a well-trained professional and have access to necessary expert resources.
7. Caseloads must be small enough to permit for needed intensity and frequency of contact.
8. Case management is an ongoing support and should, therefore, not be artificially time limited.
9. Clients need access to the case manager or familiar team members on a twenty-four hour, seven-days-a-week basis.
10. Case managers need to encourage self-determination and autonomy on the part of clients.

Home-visiting programs able to incorporate these principles are likely to engage families well and provide effective home-visiting services. In chapter 2 we will examine the ways that programs can be developed and implemented to support some of these principles. It is obvious that some of these requirements can only be met with proper funding and organizational support.

The following are some key principles typically incorporated into family-support programs for overburdened families:

1. Respect and attention are given to the family member's perspective and goals.
2. Adequate supports are provided for the family in areas of functioning in which they may be deficient. A system of support needs to be identified which will enable the family to maintain its highest level of functioning.
3. Individualized family service plans address the whole family; although problems and areas of dysfunction are taken into account, the family's ability to function independently on multiple dimensions is bolstered through a program of training and support that includes many of the environmental and contextual variables that impinge upon the family. Groups are used to help family members practice and build skills.
4. Interventions are coordinated, and fixed responsibility for the family's service plan is clearly identified. The responsibility for implementing the service plan rests with the home visitor, and the rest of the team serves to support and guide the home visitor in carrying out an effective plan for the family. The home visitor remains continuously with the family as the family moves from service system to service system in the community.
5. The program is intended to enhance the skills of all family members and encourages and accommodates growth on the part of family members.
6. It is important for family members to experience successes and movement from one level or goal to another.
7. There needs to be a focus on developing skills and competencies which will enhance the family's capacity to cope and adapt.

As a result of working with families, participating in research studies, and sharing evaluation results with colleagues in other family-support home-visiting programs, I developed an approach to providing comprehensive family-support services called Integrated Team Case Management (Carrilio 2001; 1998). In conceptualizing a model, the individual home visitor was seen as the contact point with a family, but the entire team participates in assessment, planning, and intervention. The members of the team may vary depending upon the program goals, but often include both home visitors and specialists in different areas, such as mental health, domestic violence, or substance abuse. Following the model utilized in Assertive Case Management (Stein and Santos 1998), the caseload belongs to the team and not the individual worker. There is a strong focus on developing a supportive relationship with the home visitor, with the team providing support in the form of services and resources. Other home-visiting programs may focus more on the development of a relationship with an individual case manager supervised by a skilled professional (Rapp and Goscha 2004; Heinicke et al. 2000). Supporting a psychoeducational, skill-building model (Stein and Santos 1998; Zeitz 1995; Yoshikawa 1995), center-based groups and classes were also included as key components (Carrilio 2001; Carrilio 1998). In chapters 8 and 9 the ways that teams and center-based services work in family-support home-visiting programs will be further explored.

PROGRAM PROCESS SUPPORTS OVERBURDENED FAMILIES

In working with family members to develop goals and a vision for the future, it is vital to work with the family in a way that builds upon existing strengths and leaves them feeling empowered to manage their lives. Sometimes it is hard to resist the urge to just do things for the family or to step in to fix a problem. An empowering approach:

- Focuses on the health, mental health, and developmental needs of all family members
- Focuses on the parent's health, mental health, and developmental needs
- Helps families manage risk factors
- Develops skills in the activities of daily living
- Changes negative environmental factors
- Builds community resources and social supports and teaches families to maintain and utilize these resources and supports

Empowerment refers to a focus on working as partners with families to help them identify their own strengths and solutions. An empowerment strategy is one that works with families to identify what parts of their lives they have control over, and encourages families to develop skills that will serve them in the present and in resolving future life challenges.

Some readers might be wondering if these concepts of empowerment and focusing on strengths can be utilized with child protective services cases, especially when services are not voluntary. The answer lies in the program model and clear articulation of the differences between a prevention program and an intervention program. A family-support program with involuntary clients in which both the home visitor and the family may have court-ordered requirements and constraints *can* be managed in an empowering way. To do so involves an honest acceptance of the situation by both the home visitor and the client. An empowering relationship with a client who is in the system will involve an honest appraisal of the situation and the development of a partnership to accomplish the client's goals. At its best, such a relationship helps the individual to accept the needed changes as goals of his or her own. Essentially the home visitor's task would be to help the family to internalize goals that initially may have been imposed by external agents such as the courts or child protective services.

In chapter 3, when we explore the engagement process further, it should become clear that the nature of the program will strongly affect the engagement process. Additionally, even when individuals are court ordered to carry out certain activities and tasks, approaching them in a way that offers mastery and ownership of the process is more likely to build efficacy and commitment than is an approach that relies on making the individual comply with external demands. A strengths-based empowering approach recognizes the importance of meeting the external demands, but works with the family to internalize these goals. The underlying assumption is that building efficacy reduces learned helplessness and helps to teach the individual or family coping skills that can be used in the future. Family-focused services consider the needs and goals of the family, following the philosophy that all families have strengths which can be mobilized, and the most effective strategy for empowering families is one in which they experience control over the process and are not simply passive recipients. Each family is viewed within its unique context and with its unique dynamics, and services are tailored specifically to the family's needs and goals.

Positive change in a family's life builds upon the family members' individual and collective capacities and strengths. There is an assumption that not all behavior is pathological and that the positive, healthy capacities of the family can be enhanced and supported to help the family improve its circumstances.

Many who receive family-support services have had previous negative experiences with helpers. Even the most well-intentioned helper can be perceived as harmful by a family if:

• The help provided undermines the family's sense of competence and control.
• The helper fosters dependence.
• Receiving help reduces the self-esteem of family members.
• The family feels like they "owe" the helper something.
• The help is experienced as imposed from outside and not requested by the family, harming family members' already fragile self-esteem. In cases of involuntary services,

Karla

Karla, age 22, was referred for family-support services by the hospital social worker because she had had no prenatal care, admitted to using drugs during the pregnancy, was in financial difficulty, and the social worker felt the household was chaotic. The father of the baby was in jail at the time of delivery. Karla indicated at the time of referral that she was nervous about receiving services because the home visitor would disapprove of her living situation, particularly the many acquaintances coming in and out of her apartment.

The home visitor needed to engage in active, consistent outreach, and found it very difficult to establish a regular home-visiting schedule with Karla. Home visits were inconsistent because Karla was frequently unavailable. Several weeks into the relationship, the home visitor filed a Child Protective Services report because she was concerned about the lack of bonding between Karla and baby Alex and suspected that Karla was still actively using drugs. Karla had revealed that the child was not planned and had come at a bad time in her life. The home visitor observed that normal attachment and bonding were not occurring. There was concern that the child was being neglected, especially after the home visitor learned that Karla periodically left the baby with friends so she could stay up all night on drugs.

Another report was filed two weeks later, because Karla's older child (female, age two) was left alone at home without supervision for long periods while Karla went out. The two year old had several episodes of running out into busy intersections when not being supervised.

In the same month as the reports were made to Child Protective Services, Karla was arrested for outstanding warrants. Some of these warrants were for possessing drug paraphernalia. She spent several days in jail. The local police knew her well and were in her home frequently for disturbance calls.

The child development specialist was asked to go out on a consulting home visit to observe the infant Alex, and identified concerns regarding general neglect, lack of stimulation, possible developmental delays, and possible failure to thrive. The two year old showed attachment problems and cognitive and speech delays.

---

the initial and continuing challenge will be helping the family to integrate their own wishes and dreams with the external demands.
- The help is not what the family was seeking.
- The helper provides what he/she thinks is needed, but the family may not agree.

When overburdened families have negative experiences with helpers they often start to believe that they cannot improve or change what is happening to them. This attitude is sometimes called "learned helplessness." It comes from multiple experiences in which the family member could not predict or control what was going to happen. As a result, the family member loses faith in his/her own efficacy, which is a belief in one's ability to accomplish something. A person who feels helpless often has trouble picturing a future. This makes it hard to set goals beyond the immediate resolution of the current crisis. An important part of goal setting is to reestablish hope and a sense of moving toward a future. It is important to encourage the family to think about those medium-range and long-range goals.

In setting goals with families, it is useful to keep in mind the following assumptions about families:

- Families are important; a child's primary experiences and developmental tasks are enhanced by a nurturing environment which is able to identify and meet the child's needs and to provide continuity and stability.
- In order to meet the needs of their children, parents need to be able to meet their own needs. Parents struggling with childhood trauma, or who have not had positive role models frequently need reparenting themselves, in order to develop a strong sense of identity and self-esteem so that they can better meet the needs of their children.
- Parents can develop new skills so they can understand themselves and their children better and engage in problem solving, which will improve the family's well-being.

Family-support programs utilize information about early attachment, the development of a sense of self, and the development of an internalized sense of control and structure (Heinicke et al. 2000; Carrilio 2001; Howe et al. 1999; Erikson and Kurtz-Reimer 1999; Klass 1996). While many authors explore development from their own unique perspectives, the phenomena involved in the development of the child, parent, and family unit are generally agreed to have the following characteristics:

- Movement from less structured to more structured
- Development as an ongoing process, which is continually being reworked
- Development as the establishment of internal structures that reflect both experience and the individual's reaction to the experience
- The centrality of the early parenting/holding environment in both introducing the world to children, in developing trust, and in establishing continuity and security
- Parenting as an active undertaking that requires skills and creates developmental challenges for the parent (Eisenberg and Carrilio 1983; Carrilio and Walter 1984)
- Developmental issues can be revisited at any point in the life cycle

SUMMARY

In this chapter we have examined some of the underlying principles of home visiting and case management in home-visiting programs. The reasons for developing these complex programs include:

1. Growing evidence that early childhood events and experiences can powerfully affect cognitive development, the development of substance abuse problems, criminal and violent behavior, health status, employment and life course development.
2. Increased research in a variety of fields regarding the benefits of activities that, for want of a better term, are often called "intensive case management."

■

SIDEBAR 1.6

Amelia

Nineteen-year-old Amelia was referred for family-support services by the hospital social worker. At hospital admittance for her second child, Amelia indicated that she had just been evicted and had nowhere to go when she left the hospital. Family-support services were funded by a grant to the hospital.

Amelia had been living on her own until shortly before the birth of her baby, when she was evicted. Her apartment was dirty and disorganized, and repeated complaints by other tenants led to the eviction.

The home visitor assisted Amelia in obtaining public assistance, including limited health insurance, and in making an arrangement to move back to her mother's home, a fairly stable environment. The home visitor noted that Amelia was frequently lethargic and seemed uninterested during the home visits. She seemed disconnected from the two children, and did not seem to get any joy out of their developmental progress.

Shortly after the home visitor began seeing Amelia, as part of the routine screening associated with becoming a participant in the limited publicly funded health care program, Amelia was diagnosed with lupus, a serious auto-immune disorder which can cause severe fatigue, kidney problems, heart problems, photosensitivity, rashes, severe arthritis, and other difficulties. The illness flares and then recedes, although episodes of intense symptoms can be severe. Amelia has required several hospitalizations, further disrupting her bonding with her children. The home visitor has advocated with public funding agencies to obtain funding for some of Amelia's health needs. Grandmother helps by providing childcare and managing the children's day-to-day activities, but Amelia struggles with maintaining enough energy to interact with the children regularly. The home visitor is working with Amelia and her mother to help them develop a consistent environment for the children.

3. Increased recognition of the concept of resiliency—the differential ability to thrive even under adverse circumstances has encouraged many professionals to seek ways to build protective factors and reduce vulnerability factors for families and children.

4. Recognition of an ecological perspective, which recognizes the reciprocal input into both health and dysfunction made both by the family and the larger social environment. For this reason more attention is being focused on enhancing community capacity as well as family skill building.

5. Recent brain research that identifies the vital role of the early years in the development of lifelong cognitive and emotional capacities.

6. Increased understanding of the importance of early attachment and relationship development in cognitive development and emotional regulation.

7. A frustration with, and unwillingness to accept the adverse consequences that both practice and research have associated with insufficient support to families and children during important developmental phases.

8. Humanitarian considerations and professional values that encourage us to both reduce suffering and enhance functioning along many dimensions.

TWO

Home Visiting in an Organizational Context

An organizational culture that provides adequate resources and structure for home visitors is a prerequisite to providing quality case management to vulnerable families. The home visitor needs to be embedded in an organization that offers rational, consistent, and fair policies and procedures, as well as training and professional supervision to carry out the job. Because family-support home visiting often occurs in a multiservice program context it is important that the design of the program and the way that it operates reflect the program principles. It is important to keep in mind that the purpose of these programs is to enhance family resiliency and prevent adverse outcomes (Carrilio 1998; Hall et al. 2002; Walker 2001; Guterman 2001; Shonkoff and Phillips 2000). The home visitor should have a clear understanding of how his/her activities are part of a coherent program conceptual model. When the home visitor understands the program conceptual base and the way that her role fits into the larger context, she is likely to provide more effective services to families.

Figure 2.1 Home-visiting services embedded in a multilayered systems context

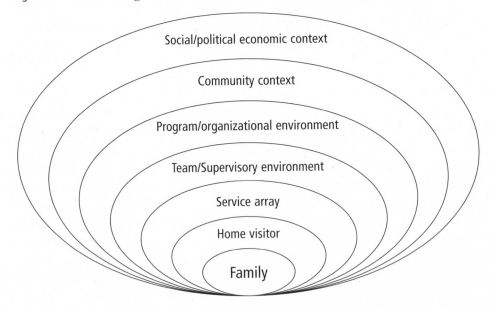

Figure 2.1 reflects an important aspect of family-support programs: home visiting is one component embedded in a larger system of care. Case management is the name often given to the "linchpin" (Weiss 1993) function that the home visitor plays. It should be clear, however, that no part of the system stands alone, and that home visiting is best nested within a system that provides support at every level. Sometimes organizations attempt to operate home-visiting programs as single, categorical programs. This happens when the organization receives funding to carry out a stand-alone program that may not be incorporated into the overall context of the organization and its mission. Effective family-support programs are best organized as part of a comprehensive system of care (Weiss 1993; O'Connor 1988). Failure to do so may compromise both the quality and effectiveness of services. In three different family-support home-visiting program initiatives, the author and colleagues had an opportunity to observe more than twenty-five home-visiting programs from initiation to the time the project was completed (Carrilio, Packard and Clapp 2003; Carrilio 2003a; Carrilio 2006). We observed that even though many program staff believe that they are following the program model, in reality implementation often falls far short of expectations (Carrilio 2005b). Additionally, even when the program is fairly well implemented, the results are mixed or weak (Sherwood 2005; Chaffin, Bonner, and Hill 2001; Culross 1999). In trying to understand our observations, we have looked at the question of whether home-visiting programs suffer from model insufficiency or failure of implementation. It may be that programs that are not well embedded in a system are not able to sustain the holistic theoretical model that underlies family-support home visitation. The day-to-day pressures and lack of consistent support from the parent organization or outside funders results in "model drift," and staff find themselves without a clear focus as they try to carry out interventions. Perhaps more concerning is the observation that many programs attempt to utilize home visiting not only as the *core* service, but also as the *only* service. While home visiting can be an important component of helping to stabilize a family and maintain progress, on its own, without a substantial case management or "linchpin" (Weiss 1993) function, or without specific interventions focused on the specific challenges facing a family, home visiting may not be as effective as its advocates proclaim.

The way the home visitor feels about the work she does, the families she works with, and herself can be strongly influenced by the organizational environment (Carrilio, Packard, and Clapp 2003; Glisson 2000; Woodside and McClam 2003).The program's underlying beliefs about the work and approach to management significantly affect the day-to-day experience of home visitors working in family-support programs. The way that a program functions day to day is influenced by the way that it was originally developed and implemented, the resource and political environment in the larger community, as well as by the beliefs of staff and administrators (Carrilio, Packard, and Clapp 2003; Clapp and Burke 1997; Straw and Herrell 2002). Figure 2.2 illustrates the ways that program implementation and outcomes are influenced by multiple factors, both internal and external to the program itself.

Figure 2.2 Influences on program operations and outcomes

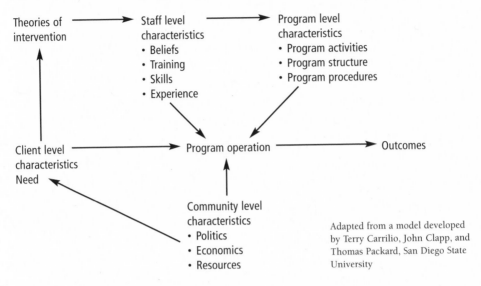

Adapted from a model developed by Terry Carrilio, John Clapp, and Thomas Packard, San Diego State University

Home-visiting programs are high risk (Sherwood 2005) in that there are often significant policy and funding implications attached to them. It is important to develop a clear understanding of the programs' purpose. For example, is it acceptable to carry out a program that supports and maintains functioning, but may not be powerful enough to reduce negative behavioral patterns such as repeated incidents of child abuse (MacMillan et al. 2005)? Heather Weiss raised this question in a discussion of the uses and effectiveness of home-visiting programs (1993). She concluded that in many vulnerable families, home visiting is *necessary* to improving family functioning and outcomes, but it may not be *sufficient,* in that the challenges facing the family, such as patterns of abuse, mental illness, or substance abuse, require more specific interventions.

PROGRAM DEVELOPMENT AFFECTS PROGRAM OPERATIONS AND OUTCOMES

Recent writers in the field of human service organizational management (Kettner 2002; Lewis et al. 2001) stress the importance of the organizational context in developing effective, high quality human services. Kettner emphasizes the need for programs to maintain internal consistency and for multiple programs and functions in an organization to function harmoniously. From the moment a program is conceptualized, through implementation, ongoing operations, and evaluation, it is important to maintain clarity of purpose and to make sure that the way things are done is consistent with this purpose. Sidebar 2.1 summarizes a process of program development, implementation, operation, and evaluation that encourages reflection and attention to quality. Most good programs follow a systematic approach to moving from the identified need, to program activities, to understanding outcomes.

The following steps are best employed at the beginning of any new program, but can also be applied as part of an ongoing process of quality management.

Phase 1: Program Concept

Family-support programs develop to meet community needs. The way these needs are defined is a function of the community's political, social, and resource context. How people understand social problems, who they feel is responsible for those problems, and the solutions they identify grow out of the shared values and experiences of the community. Ideally, once the community identifies a need among vulnerable families and key stakeholders are identified, the program development team will gather information about interventions that might be appropriate to the identified need. With the stakeholders, an intervention approach is defined and a logic model is developed. A logic model is a clear plan that describes the connections among program goals, activities, and outcomes. It is the underlying conceptual framework that helps the home

> SIDEBAR 2.1
>
> Steps in Developing and Operating Effective Programs
>
> I. Phase 1: **Program Concept**
>   A. Identify a need or problem.
>   B. Develop a program conceptual model.
>   1. Prepare a logic model.
> II. Phase 2: **Implementation**
>   A. Set organizational structure and staffing.
>   B. Develop an implementation plan and timeline.
>   1. Include a staff recruitment/retention plan.
>   2. Develop a personnel process consistent with goals values and mission set forth in the logic model.
>   3. Develop a supervision and training plan.
>   C. Develop a budget and resource plan.
>   D. Identify key internal and external stakeholders.
>   1. Develop a communications and feedback process with stakeholders.
> III. Phase 3: **Program Operations**
>   A. Develop and implement a quality management plan.
>   B. Develop and implement an information system.
> IV. Phase 4: **Program Evaluation**

visitor understand what to do and why. Once a logic model has been put forward, program implementation begins. Program implementation is the process through which the program concept, embodied in the logic model, is translated into program operations. Usually this involves coordinating staff resources and capacities with the specific interventions and theories identified in the logic model. This is a crucial part of program development.

Develop a Program Conceptual Model

A program with a strong underlying conceptual framework provides the home visitor with clear direction. Clarity of the program model can also increase the individual flexibility of the home visitor; if the underlying principles are understood and followed, there is likely to be less unnecessary focus on issues of compliance, and a reduced tendency to enforce program structures for their own sakes. Clear intervention models provide the home visitor with guidance and structure and do not need to be constraining. Rules are most rigidly enforced in circumstances in which they are seen as external and are not well integrated into practice. For this reason the home visitor and the program team would do well to focus upon articulating and clarifying the program's underlying concepts.

Many home-visiting programs recognize the importance of attachment and relationships and use concepts of efficacy and resiliency to structure their interventions. Research suggests that programs should also consider incorporating mental health and substance abuse services in planning interventions. The importance of community well-being to family well-being cannot be understated, and it is important for the program model to incorporate a focus on improving communities and their resources. The home-visiting model used by your program should be clear about how interventions will affect the problems that have been identified. The home visitor's role and the interaction of the home visitor with other team members and the community should be articulated clearly.

Prepare a Logic Model

It is often helpful for a program to prepare and share a logic model in the form of a diagram to which staff can refer. While there are many formats for creating logic models, figure 2.3 illustrates a basic model.

Developing a conceptual model and putting the model into a diagram helps to clarify the program's purpose and expectations of the home visitor *and* the families. It is also important that the logic model and conceptual model be "live" documents, in that they should be something with which all staff are familiar, and they should be reviewed and updated at regular intervals.

If your program does not have an up-to-date logic model, you can create one for yourself. You can do this by going to each box described in figure 2.3 and trying to fill it in with what you know about the program goals and the ways that specific program activities are connected to those goals. Figure 2.4 gives an example of a logic model that was used for a complex, multilayered program that incorporated family resource center activities with home visiting. While your program may not have this many elements, the diagram should give you an idea about how the program elements fit together into a coherent model.

Figure 2.3 Logic model components

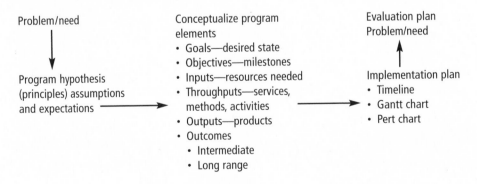

Figure 2.4 Example of a program logic model

Desired outcomes	Assumptions	Program activities	Process	Effectiveness	Impact
Families are functioning optimally Children are ready for school	All family members are developing optimally All family members are healthy Parental life course outcome move towards self sufficiency Adverse outcomes are reduced	Team case management Center-based groups and services Home visiting Information and education Child development evaluation and intervention Child-focused groups and programs Focus on life skills and problem solving	MIS data Team functioning evaluation Site surveys/interviews Standardized instruments Family service plans	Quality management checklist—items documented Family service plans regularly reviewed Use of regular assessments in service planning Case files meet standards and progresnotes reflect use of specialists and awareness of key issues from assessment Evidence of use of team through minutes, progress notes, MIS Review of group curriculum content & process	Pre/post or repeated measures Well-care compliance Early identification & intervention of risk factors Increased number of families in school or work Assess cost
Families live in safe & supportive communities	Prevention is on community agenda Resources redirected to prevention Newly designed integrated systems are sustained over time	On-going family resource center Community-wide collaboratives Training in blended funding processes and procedures Ongoing provision of comprehensive, integrated services	Funding structure and budget plans Document review Survey evaluation of collaborative efforts	Community & family feedback Review of minutes of commnity collaboratives	Identification of community challenges & strategies for change Formalized action agreements Funding plan in place

Phase 2: Implementation

An implementation plan is a description of what you will do to carry out your program, who will do it, and when it will be accomplished. Once you are familiar with the underlying program concepts and the service components that are going to make up the program, it is important to develop a plan of action that will assure that all of the necessary pieces will be put in place. One approach is to develop a "cookbook" that identifies every program element and clarifies what things would look like if the program element were to be perfectly accomplished. Sidebar 2.2 illustrates the "cookbook" for a complex family-support program that was attempting to implement a holistic vision incorporating elements at the client, staff, organizational, and community level.

Set Organizational Structure and Staffing

A key component of the implementation plan is to identify the organizational structure for the program. There are two options that most programs consider: 1) an individualistic case-management / home-visiting approach in which each staff member is assigned a caseload and in which home visitors operate independently within the parameters of organizational or program-level rules and procedures, and 2) a team approach in which a work team is assigned to manage a set of services and a given caseload. The team operates following organizational rules and procedures and establishes its own goals, quality management, and methods of assuring mutual accountability.

It is often helpful to develop organizational charts showing who is responsible for each part of the program's activities and how the different activities of the program or organization interact and support each other. Figure 2.5 shows the basic organizational chart for a team organization. This chart illustrates a structure in which the entire team is responsible for working with families.

Figure 2.5 Team organizational chart—team case management

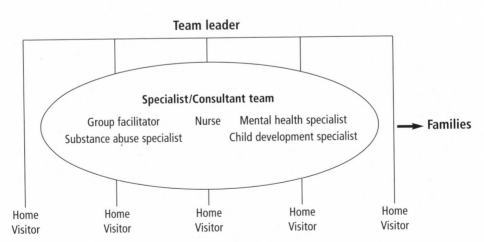

SIDEBAR 2.2

Program Model Elements—A Sample Program "Cookbook"

Model elements	Complete	Comments
1. Multidisciplinary team is staffed		
• Staffing includes:		
• Full-time, on-site team leader		
• Home visitors		
• Nurse		
• Specialists (child development, substance abuse, mental health)		
• Other:		
2. Staff training		
• Preservice training program		
• Training for team leader and specialists		
• Training for each service component		
• Regular training updates		
• Individualized training plan		
3. Supervision		
• Each team member receives individual supervision weekly minimum of one hour		
• Weekly team meetings		
• Program director provides support through:		
• supervision of team leader		
• management of policies & resources to support program		
• periodic attendance at team meeting		
• Case load is limited to 20–25 families		
4. Facility		
• Adequate workspace for each team member		
• Meeting space for team is available		
• Rooms for groups and childcare are available		
• Facility meets local code standards and ADA standards		
• Private areas are available to meet with clients		
• Phone, computer, communications technology available to staff		
5. Program Activities/Services		
• Team case management approach		
• Use of standardized screening and assessment tools		
• Clearly defined target population		
• Logic model connects services to goals		
• Service plan developed and implemented within 30 days of service initiation		
• Service plan is clearly connected to the assessment		

SIDEBAR 2.2 (*continued*)

Model elements	Complete	Comments
• Regular progress notes and reevaluation of plan		
• Home-visiting content set by service plan		
• Clear transportation policy		
• Clearly articulated group program with a regular schedule		
• Group curriculum consistent with population needs		
• Registration and attendance policies set for groups		
6. Quality Management		
• Regular review of program goals and consistency of services with goals		
• Regular utilization review		
• Structured information system used by all staff		
• Case record system that clearly documents consent, health status, assessments, service plans, and progress notes		
• Emergency plans in place		
• Safety plans exist and are updated regularly		
• Measure the gap between services as planned and services as delivered		
• Case notes are done after each contact and are clear, concise, and based on observations		
• Process data is entered regularly and staff receive performance feedback		
• Strategic plan is in place and is regularly reviewed and updated		
• Program operates with a clear logic model and implementation plan		
• Implementation and operations plan account for resources and barriers		
• Regular review of policies and procedures to assure support for program model		
7. Governance and Policies		
• Personnel policies are clear, consistent with best practices, and updated regularly		
• Written mission statement		
• Clear organizational chart		
• Governing body evidences support and regularly monitors program		
• Progress reports are provided to the governing body on a regular basis		
• Governing body has the authority to plan, utilize resources, assess program services, oversee the program		
• Governing body is familiar with program budget and resources		
• Governing body is responsible for personnel procedures as well as all policies and procedures of the organization, reviewed regularly, in cooperation with program staff		

Developed by Terry Carrilio, Beth Sheffield, and Malia Adler, Social Policy Institute at San Diego State University

Another component of the program structure and organization has to do with caseload size. If team case management is decided upon, there will need to be a sense of how many families can be managed by a single team. If individual home visitor case management is decided upon, there will need to be an understanding of how many families each home visitor can effectively manage. It is suggested that caseloads for individual home visitors be maintained at twenty to twenty-five families. A team with five home visitors and several specialists can effectively manage 100–125 families.

Another decision will involve the use of shared resources among teams. It may be effective to share specialists, such as nurses, child development specialists, group coordinators, mental health specialists, and substance abuse specialists between two teams. However, it will be important to establish structures that will protect these shared staff from overutilization. Additionally the staff shared across teams should have its own reference group. For example, substance abuse specialists should be able to meet and receive training and support regularly. This enables the specialty staff to stay up to date, obtain support, and provides an opportunity for reflection on the group processes occurring in the teams.

Implementation Plan with Timeline

The implementation plan should also include a way of keeping track of all of the activities and illustrate the flow and timing of these activities. Many programs utilize simple timelines or flow charts to show what activities will take place and when they will occur. The GANTT chart is a simple way to list program implementation activities and keep track of who will carry them out (Lewis et al. 2001, 64). Figure 2.6 is an example of the GANTT chart for a sample home-visiting program. There are a number of other simple ways to prepare implementation plans. Some program developers prefer PERT charts, or Management by Objectives models (Lewis et al. 2001). In any case the implementation plan should clearly follow from the program's conceptual model and should make it clear how the program elements needed to satisfy the logic model will be put into place. The idea is to find a simple way to identify all of the activities that need to take place in order to begin the program and to think through when and how they will take place. The timeline serves as an excellent template for a quality management plan as well, since it allows staff, supervisors, and administrators to quickly identify activities and monitor progress.

Staff Recruitment/Retention Plan

As part of implementation, it is important to identify the type of staff and the number required to meet the requirements of the program conceptual model. Programs vary widely in the educational and experiential expectations of home visitors. Some programs, such as HIPPY, PAT, and Healthy Families, utilize community-based paraprofessionals, and often family members themselves, while others utilize professional nurses or social workers (Heinicke et al. 2000; Olds et al. 2002). Different levels of training and experience will affect the amount and type of supervision home visitors

Figure 2.6 Sample GANTT chart (first year of new program implemetation and operation)

Activity	Month 1	Month 2	Month 3	QTR 2	QTR 3	QTR 4
Startup planning						
• Hire project director	▓	▓	▓			
• Hire team leader	▓					
• Hire administrative assistant	▓	▓	▓			
• Identify MIS • Purchase hardware and software			▓			

• Obtain Facility
  • Purchase furnishings and Equipment
  • Set up phone system
		▓	▓			

• Prepare a policies and procedures manual		▓	▓			
• Develop emergency plans		▓				
• Introduce project to community			▓			
Staff recruitment and training						
Client recruitment and screening				▓	▓	
Home visits				▓	▓	▓
Group and classes						
• Develop curriculum, policies, and procedures		▓	▓			
• Develop a transportation plan		▓	▓			
Quality reviews						
• Review records		▓	▓			
• Ongoing MIS reports					▓	▓
Progress reports to board/administration/community				▓	▓	▓

need, and will affect the content of the training program. It is important that the staff are hired in a systematic way, and that qualifications be tied to the program concept and the activities that staff are expected to perform. The training and experience of the home visitors chosen for a particular program will affect the level of oversight and degree of autonomy permitted. A program with trained, licensed social workers or psychologists will be more likely to permit autonomy, with the understanding that the professional is acting in accordance with the program's underlying conceptual principles. On the other hand, a program using paraprofessional or indigenous staffing would need to provide more direct guidance and oversight of home visitor activities.

The staffing structure suggested in figure 2.5 requires support and resources from the parent organization. Staff need to be trained and supported in their roles. Team leaders need support and training in order to manage the group process of the team. With shared staff, the additional dynamic introduced by having group members who are not "owned" by the group will need attention. By focusing on these important support and group dynamics considerations, a program developer can do much to improve morale and staff retention.

Personnel Process

A key component of retention and of quality implementation has to do with the way personnel policies and procedures are carried out. It is here that the concept of "parallel process" becomes real. If staff are treated fairly, consistently, and predictably, it is likely that they will be better able to provide the kind of support and consistency needed by overburdened families. Conversely, personnel processes that are experienced as disempowering by the home visitors may make it difficult for them to work with families in a way that is consistent with program goals and philosophy.

Supervision and Training Plan

Working with vulnerable families is difficult and personally challenging. Many families can bring up issues and unresolved dynamics for the home visitor and other team members. Good supervision and training are essential to helping the home visitor to maintain a professional stance with families. Weekly supervision of all home visitors and team members is essential, as is an opportunity for the team to meet jointly. These team meetings serve to coordinate activities and identify areas for further training. In chapter 10 the use and functioning of teams in family-support home-visiting programs will be examined.

Training involves both understanding the overall perspective of the program as well as the development of specific skills. The training program will need to be geared to the education and experience of the home-visiting staff. Professionals, such as social workers or psychologists, are likely to be licensed and to have a good understanding of ethics, professional boundaries, and the structure of interviews. Although they will need to learn about the specific expectations of the program, there would probably be more focus on the conceptual basis of the program and opportunities for the home visitor to work through examples of its application. Paraprofessionals and indigenous home visitors may require more information about boundaries, ethics, systems, and self-care. At this level more direct supervision will be required in order to assure that program activities are consistent with the program's conceptual model.

It is important for staff skills to be current and relevant to the specific aims of the program. For instance, if your home-visiting program focuses on school readiness as one of its key organizing principles, staff training should include general information about child development as well as specific information about helping parents to build cognitive and social skills. It is suggested that home visitors receive an intensive pre-service training that orients them to the organization and to the program's conceptual model, and offers specific operational guidelines and general information about key topics such as child development, attachment, communications skills, language development, family routines, play, cultural diversity, and age-appropriate discipline.

The specific training program established by a home-visiting program will depend heavily on its underlying conceptual model, logic model, and implementation plan. In short the training needs to specifically prepare home visitors to meet the goals and expectations of the particular program in which they are working. While there may be a great deal of carryover from one program to another, it is important that training be specifically tailored to the program goals and that staff receive sufficient training and support in operational and procedural considerations so that they are fully prepared to function in a specific program and organizational context.

Preservice training assures that home visitors understand the program context and content. Many programs choose to develop a training manual that includes key procedural and conceptual information. This manual is useful to the home visitor and the supervisor, helping to structure the work and providing useful reference information. Once the initial preservice training has been completed, the home visitor and supervisor should regularly assess training needs and establish a training plan. Some programs carry out regular monthly or bimonthly training programs, while others may work with individual home visitors to identify training and skill-building opportunities. It is important to assure that there is a program of ongoing training to build and maintain the home visitor's skills and knowledge.

Budget and Resource Plan

Key to the functioning of any program are adequate financial resources. While this may seem entirely self-evident, it is unfortunately the case that many family-support programs function on shoe-string budgets and may not have sufficient resources to allocate to the task at hand. Kettner (2002) points out that budgeting has not always been a focus in human services agencies. Often administrators, staff, and community members have focused on the importance of the organization's mission and the value-based approval of the organization's activities. Human service organizations have an ability to function in the absence of good budget information and budget management that would not be tolerated or even possible in the business world (Kettner). Never the less, effective budget management and re-source allocation is essential for program effectiveness and quality.

When the author was in graduate school, one of the truisms that was repeated over and over again was that "form follows finance." This essentially means that financial resources strongly influence the way an organization functions and is structured. This seems obvious, but surprisingly, many human service administrators and staff substitute attention to the "good" that is being done for attention to the way in which the funding structure, resource allocation, and resource management affect the program. The way that financial resources are applied and managed can support or inhibit program functioning in a way that goes beyond mere dollars and cents. It is important to assure that the resources needed in order to carry out the program are available. For instance, the resources to assure a facility that is clean, safe, and adequate for offices, group, and center-based operations are a prerequisite to operating a multiservice family-support program. Yet, in many instances, because of inadequate resources, program staff are not provided with the facilities needed to do the job.

A more serious concern has to do with managing and allocating resources such that staff are adequately compensated and that the personnel policies reflect the philosophy of support and autonomy that family-support programs attempt to engender. Sidebar 2.3 describes a case history of how form follows finance. It should be clear from this example that although home-visiting services were being offered by this agency, family support was *not* being offered. The families being served in such a manner are likely to feel like cogs in a machine, and they are probably not going to experience a restorative, supportive

---

SIDEBAR 2.3

Form Follows Finance
Case #1: New Vistas

The New Vistas Family Support Program was part of a large community nonprofit organization that had been operating in Metroville for over twenty years. After a competitive bidding process, New Vistas obtained a contract from the county to provide prevention and early intervention services to families at risk of child abuse. The families were referred by community agencies or through the child welfare agency that had investigated the case and found that the family was not currently at a risk level necessitating child welfare services. The structure of the funding was such that New Vistas would be paid for only home visits completed. No-shows, groups, outreach, and case management, while implicit in the contract, were not set as contract goals, and were not reimbursed. New Vistas was also provided with funds to offer two parenting classes. Statistics for the parenting classes and home visiting were to be kept separately; home-visiting clients were not expected to attend the classes, and payment for the classes was based solely on the number of sessions held and the maintenance of a minimal enrollment.

Sally H. was hired as a home visitor to work on this contract. She received no formal training and was handed a manual of forms and procedures on her first day. Her supervisor limited contact to making sure billing forms and backup materials in the case file were complete. Sally was hired for fifteen hours a week, so she received no benefits. Her pay rate was only slightly above the minimum wage. Her mileage, if accurately documented to the supervisor's satisfaction, could be reimbursed. Most weeks there were several dollars of "disallowances" deducted from her submitted reimbursement claim.

Sally was given a caseload of thirty-five to forty families. Her supervisor indicated that she knew that Sally would only be able to see about a third of the families because of no-shows, and suggested that Sally double book in order to maximize her salary,

(Continued next page)

since she would only be paid for home visits completed. Sally spent twenty-five to thirty hours a week working in order to make ten–twelve home visits. She was not paid for phone calls or any follow-up referrals or case management, so over time she reduced these activities to a minimum. She was paid for ten–twelve hours of work. She referred some of her clients to the parenting groups but did not spend much time following up in order to maximize the time that she had available to organize and conduct home visits.

Sally found herself avoiding challenging families because they either took too much time or would not show for appointments. She began to cut her home visits to fifty and then forty-five minutes because she could still get paid for the hour and would be able to squeeze in one or two more families in a day.

relationship over time with a skilled and effective home visitor. Even if Sally, our home visitor in this example, were highly dedicated and skilled, the funding structure and poor allocation of resources in her program would influence her ability to provide high quality family-support home visitation. Noteworthy, too, is the separation of the home-visiting and case-management functions. In this case, because the funding structure did not explicitly value the case-management component of the service, it was not valued by the organization.

It is important to note that in the above example the same funding structure could have been managed differently with a bit of administrative commitment. Sidebar 2.4 offers a case example of an organization that had obtained the same contract as New Vistas but chose to allocate its resources differently. The home visitor in case #2 averaged twenty to twenty-five home visits weekly and the organization was able to maintain a supportive infrastructure for staff with the same funding structure as in case #1. The main difference between these two approaches had to do with the existence of a conceptual model in case #2 such that the form of the program utilized the funding structure to meet the program's larger conceptual goals, while in case #1, the funding completely defined the program in the absence of a larger conceptual foundation.

Identify Key Internal and External Stakeholders
An important key to program implementation has to do with engaging stakeholders. These are the people who care what happens to the families and to the program. Stakeholders include boards of directors, other programs in an organization, other organizations, families, public agencies, schools, and, of course, the families. Funding agencies, researchers, policy makers, and others interested in family-support programs are often included among the stakeholders. It is important to identify who has an interest in the program and to enlist as much support as possible from these stakeholders. In order to do this, stakeholders need to be involved and to be aware of what is happening in the program.

Develop a Communications and Feedback Process with Stakeholders
Each type of stakeholder will need to be communicated with differently. For instance, boards of directors rely on reports and budget updates to understand how programs are doing. They are also interested in case examples and in community feedback about the program. It is important to keep boards and organizational administrators focused

Form Follows Finance—Case #2: The Family Support Center

The Family Support Center was a small program in a large organization that had developed home visiting as a volunteer community service and was seen by the parent organization and the community as an important contribution to good relations. When the request for proposals for a new home-visiting program came out, there was a great deal of debate about whether to "professionalize" and expand the services. The organization decided to apply for funding with the understanding that the program would develop a strong conceptual model and operate quality services. The Family Support Center received a contract for the same services described in case #1 in another part of Metroville. The funding structure was identical, in that the Family Support Center would only receive reimbursement for home visits actually delivered and for two group sessions to be held continuously over the course of the project. In short the Family Support Center and New Vistas were being paid the same amount and in the same manner for delivering two specific services: home visits and parenting groups.

Barbara C., a staff member at the parent agency, was asked to serve as the project director for the new contract. Barbara and her supervisor developed a conceptual model that focused on the need for families to be seen immediately in order to reduce the possibility of increased risk and on the idea that family support begins at the moment of referral. Barbara received permission from the organization to hire a team leader, three full-time home visitors, and an administrative support person. These staff members would receive benefits and would be placed in the salary structure of the larger parent organization, giving them a career ladder. Barbara and the new team leader decided that it would be vital to conduct parenting groups in order to enhance continuity, allow parents to practice new skills, and maintain contact with new families who had not yet developed a strong relationship with a home visitor. Barbara and the team leader conducted two groups a week, in English and Spanish, and obtained support from the parent organization to pay a transportation company to bring families to the groups. Part-time childcare aides were hired and home visitors rotated responsibility for assisting with the childcare.

The home-visiting team met weekly and the home visitors and childcare aides received individual supervision weekly. Home visitors were encouraged to work holistically with their families and to provide the referrals and case management needed to meet the family-support goals of the program. The clerical staff person utilized an information system to track contacts and worked closely with the project director and team leader to track the number of home visits and group sessions that could be billed to the funder. The project director and team leader understood that in order to afford the staffing and infrastructure they had put in place, a certain number of home visits were required monthly. However, home visitors were encouraged to focus on the needs of the families and were only advised of a need to increase home-visiting contacts if the monthly number dropped below a threshold.

Vera J. was hired as a home visitor on this contract. She received one week of formal preservice training and weekly individual supervision. Vera attended weekly team meetings where cases were discussed and team members assisted each other with resources and problem solving. Issues related to the groups were raised at the team meetings. Strategies for problem solving were identified and regularly followed by the team. Vera was assigned to work with twenty-five families. She saw most of her families weekly and referred all of them to the groups. Twenty of her families attended regularly, and Vera would meet with them briefly before the group meetings to check in and offer some quick case management and follow-up. The team leader encouraged Vera to engage all of her families and worked closely with her to address issues raised by challenging families.

on the program, its purposes, its value to the organization, and the role it plays in meeting the organization's mission. Communicating with families can take place in the course of program participation through special events and periodic feedback meetings, as well as through newsletters, brochures, fliers, and e-mails. Likewise, a plan for communicating with each group of stakeholders is an important part of the program in that it maintains focus on the purpose and helps to provide resources. Program continuity may be affected by the depth and breadth of stakeholder involvement and support. There are many creative ways to maintain engagement by stakeholders. While each individual home visitor may not be in a position to manage the communication plan, each home visitor should be aware of key stakeholders in the program and have an idea about the way the program is keeping those stakeholders engaged.

Phase 3: Program Operations

Develop and Implement a Quality Management Plan

Building on the implementation plan, an operations plan should be devised. This document builds upon both the implementation plan and the logic model and provides a way for the home visitor, supervisor, and program administrator to assure that program activities are taking place as specified by the program's conceptual model. The quality management plan offers a way to review program activities and evaluate their effectiveness.

The quality management plan provides a framework for staff at all levels to identify activities that need to occur as well as to explore whether the activities are being carried out in the best way possible. A family-support program built on trust and collaboration will encourage staff to identify procedural and practical problems and review them with an eye toward improving program practices. The quality management plan looks at what is happening and compares it to what staff and stakeholders think should be happening. The gap is studied and strategies to bring actual operations closer to the ideal are developed. Once strategies for improvement are identified and implemented, the team reviews and evaluates how well they are working and makes adjustments as needed.

It should be clear from the discussion about quality management that it requires strong organizational support. In order for the home visitor and his/her team to carry out an effective quality management plan, they need to be operating in an organization that fosters self-reflection, effectiveness, and trust (Kettner 2002; Johnson and Johnson, 2006). In an atmosphere that does not support exploration of mistakes and areas in which the program needs to improve, staff may become defensive or indifferent.

Develop and Implement an Information System

In order to track quality and effectiveness it is important to think about which data need to be collected and how these data will be gathered, analyzed, and utilized. A discussion of the way that the home visitor interacts with this data system can be found in chapter 10. Oftentimes home visitors and other stakeholders find information gathering tedious. Even a very good data system, without support throughout the organizational system and subsystems, will be ineffective (Carrilio 2005a). The program developer of any home-visiting program needs to carefully plan for collecting data that demonstrates what is happening, how much is happening, who is receiving services, who is providing services, how well services are being conducted, and what results can be attributed to the program effort.

Phase 4: Program Evaluation

Kettner (2002) differentiates among factors that go into service delivery and the end results or outcomes. It is important to look at structural, organizational, and contextual factors that influence service quality and accuracy. It is important to distinguish which elements of organizational culture and context influenced service delivery behaviors in order to understand outcomes. These are the end results, and they represent all of the goals and objectives that are contained in the program's conceptual model. Because of the highly charged nature of evaluation in home-visiting programs (Stratham and Holtermann 2004; Hahn et al. 2005; Daro 2005; Sherwood, 2005), it is vital that programs do as much as possible to distinguish between implementation failures and conceptual insufficiency.

It is important to connect the program theory with outputs and outcomes in order to better understand how complex, multifaceted interventions achieve their effects (Hernandez 2000; Orwin 2000; Jerrel and Ridgely 1999). Most evaluations presume that the program was implemented, without significant variation, as designed and conceptualized. However, this may not always be the case. The clarity of the program model and the context within which evaluations occur influences how they are conducted (Simmel 2002; Leff and Mulkern 2002; Orwin 2000; Vinson 2001). An additional component to understanding program effectiveness involves not only the degree to which the program as designed was implemented, but the quality of the program that was delivered (Proctor 2002; Sluyter 1998). Implementation is a key component of program quality. Organizational context has a strong effect on how a program is implemented and operated (Moore 1998).

Often evaluators are asked to determine if a program "works." This type of question assumes a "black box" approach (Harachi et al. 1999; Donaldson and Scriven 2003). In evaluations utilizing experimental designs there is an assumption that a standardized intervention has been delivered in equal doses over the same duration of time to a treatment group. The treatment group is then compared to a control group that did not receive services from the program. It is assumed that if the intervention worked, differences between the intervention and the control group will occur. This approach to evaluation does not take into account the context of implementation, the capacity or ideology of the implementing organization, or the dimension of service quality (Jerrell and Ridgely 1999; Vinson 2001; Teague 1998; Domitrovich and Greenberg 2000). The "black box" approach has been criticized because it fails to address the elements of a program that are effective (Harachi et al. 1999; Donaldson and Scriven

2003; Domitrovich and Greenberg 2000; Vinson 2001; Carrilio 2005a). Evaluators are now moving beyond the question of "did it work?," and are beginning to explore "how?," "why?," "for whom?," and "under what circumstances do programs function?" (Harachi et al. 1999; Mark 2003; Orwin 2000).

Most evaluations do not take into account how resources, staff training and beliefs, and management affect program implementation. Yet program implementation is highly affected by the context within which the program exists as well as by ideological factors at the program administrator and staff levels (Carrilio, Packard, and Clapp 2003; Clapp and Burke 1997; Straw and Herrell 2002; Everhart and Wandersman 2000; Orwin, 2000). Without carefully considering and measuring the factors that influence levels of implementation, an evaluation's utility can be severely limited. This is a threat to science-based program design and the development of applied knowledge in human services. Additionally program staff need data about the specifics of program implementation in order address the quality of services (Proctor 2002).

SUMMARY

This chapter explores the ways in which the organizational context within which a home-visiting program is developed and implemented affects the program's quality and effectiveness. The chapter will be of interest to program directors and supervisors as they develop family-support home-visiting programs. There is a relationship between program outcomes and a clear program conceptualization. A four-phase model for program development is offered, with specific pointers for systematically carrying out each phase.

THREE

Getting Started

In this chapter we will look at the beginning stages of working with families. This chapter will be of particular interest to home visitors and their supervisors. It presents detailed information about the initial contact and engagement process with families. During this stage the home visitor will focus on engaging and setting the stage for mutuality in the relationship. Self-reflection and appropriate use of supervision are especially important.

The following diagram depicts the family-support case-management process, highlighting the first step of the case-management process.

Figure 3.1 Getting started

Family-Support Home-Visiting Case-Management Process

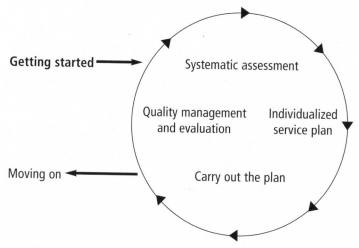

Getting started involves meeting and engaging the family in a relationship focused on growth and development. In this chapter we will be looking at the following aspects of the initial contact with a family: 1) the referral; 2) planning for the first visit; 3) the visit.

THE REFERRAL

One of the first things to consider during the beginning stage of contact is how your program recruits families into the program. Some programs recruit families based on specific risk factors, while others provide more universal services. Risk-based programs tend to identify a population based on certain characteristics, such as being poor, single, young, suffering from mental illness, substance abuse, or being at risk of child abuse or domestic violence. A universal recruitment approach would provide services to all families (for instance, in a geographic area, all new mothers in an area, and so on) without sifting with respect to risk. Universal services tend to be less stigmatizing, since everyone in a particular group is eligible for the program, regardless of risk.

The relationship with the family begins as soon as you receive a referral. It is perfectly normal that the family will be initially reticent, and if not suspicious, certainly cautious, about opening themselves up to a new relationship. In the early stages the family is sizing you up and assessing their own willingness to put energy into a new relationship. Try to find out very early in the contact with a family what their initial experience with your organization or the referral source was like. You may need to give the family time to vent and to work through what happened to them in the process of getting to you. Your willingness to listen in a nondefensive manner, especially if the family's initial experiences have been difficult, will be a first step towards building trust.

There are a number of things to consider right at the start:

1. Are You Working with a Team?

Organizations providing home-visiting and case-management services differ tremendously in their scope and organization. It is important for you to know if you are solely responsible for work with the family or if you will be sharing responsibility with other professionals and paraprofessionals. If you are part of a team providing family-support services to families, make sure you understand each team member's role and function. Work with your team and supervisor to clarify boundaries and expectations.

If you are the sole practitioner working with the family, make sure that you are clear about why the family has been referred to you and what your agency expects you to do in your work with families.

2. Do You Understand Your Program's Logic Model?

In chapter 1 the idea that family-support programs operate with an underlying theory of change was explored. Before engaging with a family, review your program's logic model. What are the goals your program is trying to achieve? What activities are part of the program, and how do these relate to the goals? How will you be tracking your activities so you can measure goal accomplishment? How much structure in the form of guidelines, training, and program curricula is available to you? Check with your supervisor to make sure you understand what services and activities you are expected to carry out, and clarify any questions you have about why certain procedures are in place. You are the program's representative in the community, so it is important for you to understand what the program is all about and how the services offered are related to the program's goals. The more clear you are about this, the easier it will be to explain to families and other community members as you work to engage them in the process of family support.

3. Do You Have Someone (Usually a Supervisor) with Whom to Review the Case?

If you are part of a team, make sure you are prepared to review your experiences with the family with your team members for the purpose of receiving guidance, support, suggestions, information, and general feedback. Be prepared to use the resources of your team and/or your supervisor to help you think through problems, questions, and concerns you have as you work with the family. Before you begin with the family, make sure you have clarified expectations with your supervisor, and make sure you are prepared to work collaboratively with your supervisor to review assessment information, concerns, and questions as they arise. Because many overburdened families present some complex concerns, it is important to remember that you are not a "lone wolf" working on the case; collaboration and creative problem solving with the family and your colleagues are an important part of assuring that the family's needs are identified and addressed. As you begin work with each family, it is a good idea to review your own resources, including the availability of a supervisor, team, and colleagues. This is a good time to refresh and revitalize the organizational relationships that support you in doing a good job with families.

4. Have You Received Any Training That Can Help You Work with the Family?

In addition to understanding the theoretical foundation and logic model of your program, you should feel confident that you know how to carry out the activities the program has asked you to carry out. Many family-support programs offer initial and ongoing training in parenting, attachment, child development, risk assessment, and other areas that come up in working with overburdened families. It is also important that you become familiar with the cultural norms and expectations of the populations your program serves. Many family-support programs provide training and other supports to help staff develop and maintain culturally competent practice. Understanding the bases of cultural and bicultural identity formation and ways in which cultural resources can provide needed supports to a family are essential. While some families will be similar to you culturally, racially, or ethnically, there are two important things to remember: 1) Similarities can hide differences in the sense that you may assume that the family shares your views or attitudes because they are from a similar background. It is vital that you put your assumptions aside and make sure to be open to hearing the family's unique perspective. 2) Being different from a family may offer you and the family an opportunity to explore some of the underlying assumptions they apply to their daily decision making. This can be wonderful chance to help the family integrate some of their values and understand how they can work with their own values and beliefs to improve their situation.

5. Do You Have Any Referral Information?

As you prepare to meet and engage the family it is helpful to review the intake information you have available. This will tell you a little about who the family is, who is in the family, and what some of their concerns might be. It also gives you information about where the family lives and the resources and other organizations with which they are involved. Simple things like knowing the family's address can also help you plan your home visits by giving you an idea of how close the family lives to other families you might be working with and how much time it will take to travel to and from your visits.

It is important to get as much information as possible regarding the referral, review any risk assessments which have already been done, and develop some questions that will help you better understand the family's needs and current situation. Although some preliminary information may help you to frame some questions or areas to assess further, it is important to avoid prejudging the situation, the family's needs, or the services the family may need and want.

The referral information will probably give you an idea about whether the family is voluntary or mandated. It is important to recognize that even families who are seeking services voluntarily may be ambivalent and hesitant to engage. Do not assume that because a family is voluntary that they are immediately ready to dive into a relationship and start working. While the reluctance of the mandated family is more understandable, all families are going to be a bit guarded and hesitant at the beginning of the relationship. Many home visitors are quite surprised to learn that their "voluntary" family forgets visits, can be hard to motivate, and takes a very long time to incorporate new learning into their daily activities. The process of engaging the family, whether they are voluntary or mandated, is key to establishing a relationship. Without developing a relationship and building some basic trust with the family, the home visitor cannot be effective in supporting family growth.

Clients who are mandated may exhibit reluctance about meeting you. Respectfully acknowledge their concerns and remain focused on establishing a space, time, and structure within which to meet. Even if the client does not initially cooperate, working toward developing a sense of your time together having boundaries of time and structure will encourage family members to respond to the consistency and continuity of their relationship with you. Remember, too, that involuntary clients do not have to accept the services of your agency, and it is not a personal insult if they continue to hesitate or otherwise avoid making a commitment

PLANNING THE FIRST VISIT

As you prepare to meet the family for the first time, think about the family's situation and try to imagine what you would feel and how you would react in a similar situation. Prior to meeting the family it is important for you to be aware of the assumptions that may be built in to the recruitment or referral process. Be honest with yourself. The more you are able to identify the stereotypes and assumptions that may be built in to the recruitment or referral process, the easier it will be for you to engage the family on a person-to-person basis. Often the information you have from a referral source or from the recruitment criteria of your program can lead to negative stereotyping and "labeling." This means that you are in danger of seeing the client in terms of labels such as the following:

- Depressed parent
- Inadequate parent
- Substance abuser
- Domestic violence victim
- Poor
- Uneducated
- Criminal
- Child abuser
- Domestic violence perpetrator
- Homeless

While the family may, in fact, be struggling with one or more of these challenges, it is important to normalize things by remembering that even people struggling with serious problems are regular people a good part of the time. This means that even people experiencing serious problems want to be engaged in a dialogue with you, as opposed to being talked down to or "talked at." Developing skills in entering dialogue with the family requires careful self-reflection and requires you to be able to both set limits and be open to the client's perspective.

In preparation for your first contact, you might want to imagine yourself in the family's situation. How would you respond to a stranger coming to your home? For many families, it is very distressing to feel they may be doing things incorrectly, and they may feel it is important for you to acknowledge any positive efforts they have made already (including agreeing to participate in a family-support home-visiting program). It is important for the family to feel that you respect them and are not coming in to tell them what they have been doing "wrong."

Often the parents in overburdened families have had developmental experiences and traumas that result in problems maintaining both trust and continuity. What this means is that they are used to starting things, running into barriers, and then ending their efforts. Over time this can lead to a profound sense of hopelessness, in that the

SIDEBAR 3.2

Preparing for the First Contact with a Family

- Think about what you would be feeling and thinking in a similar situation. What would you be worried about? What things would you be hoping to achieve?
- Even if things look bleak, most families really do want things to improve, but may not have a picture of what an improved world would look like. Your willingness to engage with them and work toward a vision for the future reinforces motivation and positive efforts.
- The family may be deciding for themselves if things are completely hopeless or if they can commit to efforts to change. There may be a great deal of ambivalence about this; on the one hand, family members may want things to be different, but on the other, the risks and discomforts of the change process are daunting. Do not assume that people are ready to jump right in and begin a change process.
- The family needs to "feel you out." They need to determine whether you seem to understand their concerns, have anything to offer, and can support them through what may be a difficult process. Essentially the family, in making a commitment to work with you, is "hiring" you to help them achieve a goal. They need to know that you are going to treat them professionally, with respect, and are going to follow through.
- You do not need to collect all of the information on your agency's intake form, or answer all of your own assessment questions immediately. Your first task is to open a dialogue with the family and determine if, in fact, they have chosen you to work with them. Once the family commits itself to begin working on some of the issues that have brought them to the attention of your organization, it is important to engage them as partners in the data-gathering effort that will enable you to jointly assess the situation and identify strategies to address it.
- Maintain some perspective on your role with the family. Remember, they will only see you for a brief time (often once or twice a week), and they will be relying on their own skills and resources most of the time. Your role is to provide them with support, resources, and information that bolsters their own problem-solving capacities, always keeping in mind that your goal is to gradually transfer more and more control and responsibility to the family to the extent that family members are prepared to manage things.

parent has little confidence that anything he or she does will work. It is important for you to maintain a sense of purpose and focus from the beginning that will allow the family to begin experiencing small successes and, more important, a sense that their efforts fall into a coherent whole.

Before meeting with the family for the first time you will also want to remind yourself of your program's health and safety procedures and follow them carefully. Make sure you have reviewed safety procedures with your supervisor, and use good judgment as you move about in the community. Most programs have developed procedures to help keep staff safe out in the field. Make sure the receptionist or another staff person knows where you are and has your cellular phone number. Have some prearranged signals to alert the program if you are having a problem while on a home visit. If you are concerned about a home for any reason, ask another staff member to accompany you.

In addition to being safety conscious, you will need to pay attention to health and cleanliness considerations. This is sometimes difficult because it is important to be careful and at the same time avoid insulting the family. It is important for you to remember that you are not judging the family by maintaining good sanitary practices, but are protecting yourself so you will not contract an illness that might prevent you from spending time with the family. Make sure your immunizations are up to date, and if available, obtain a flu shot. Some programs provide immunizations for hepatitis. Some home visitors struggle with balancing the need to be health conscious with a concern about insulting the family. Another way to look at things is to recognize that your own focus on healthy practices can be a teaching opportunity. Some home visitors develop a ritual with the family of washing their hands at the beginning and end of the visit, encouraging the family to recognize that the home visitor is also protecting their health by not carrying germs from another home into their home.

If possible, sit on plastic or wood and avoid fabric furniture. Unfortunately lice, fleas, and other unwanted organisms can reside in fabric. Pay attention to where you leave purses or briefcases (although these are best left in your trunk or at the office), since unwanted pests can enter them while you are in the home. Before having close contact with children or other family members, find out if they have something contagious such as pink eye, scabies, impetigo, lice, and so on. If someone in the home is sick, avoid contact, and, using your judgment, reschedule the visit. If you bring toys or other items into the home, make sure they are disinfected. It is often difficult for

---

SIDEBAR 3.3

Home Visitor Safety Tips

- Be sure to have a well-maintained car, and you have gas in the car.
- Be aware of any weather conditions that might affect your travel.
- Do not leave your car open, and avoid having items visible on the seats. Do not carry valuables openly in your car. If you are carrying things to bring to clients' homes, such as diapers, toys, or groceries, keep them locked in the trunk.
- Have items for your visit with you in the car, not in the trunk. (This is not a contradiction with the point above. Between visits make sure you know what you need for each family and stop at a gas station, shopping center, or other safe place in between visits to put the things you need for the next visit in the car with you.)
- Leave your purse in the office. Carry a driver's license and a small amount of cash in a pocket. If you cannot leave your purse safely in the office, lock it in your trunk. Consider using a car alarm or wheel-locking device.
- Drive safely and wear your seat belt.
- Wear a name badge if possible and introduce yourself as being from the program for which you work.
- Keep calm and confident. Make eye contact and acknowledge the presence of people nearby and in the home. Make sure you know who is in the home while you are there.
- Leave if you see excessive activity, a rapid change in behavior, unprovoked anger, open drug use, or anything else that worries you about your safety. Be alert for body language that is threatening. Follow your instincts and do not stay if you are uncomfortable.
- Wear casual, yet professional clothing. It is important not to be too "dressed up" or too "dressed down."
- Be alert. Do not leave your car in an isolated spot and pay attention to where you are when you are walking.

(Continued next page)

- Be aware of stores, churches, and other places that might be safe should you run into a problem.
- Make sure someone in the office knows where you are and the approximate length of time you expect to be there. Review your program safety procedures.
- Carry a cellular phone that is charged, and make sure your emergency numbers and contacts are preprogrammed and easily accessible.
- Plan your route in advance to avoid wandering around in an unfamiliar area. Use the restroom before leaving the office. If you are out on visits all day, make sure you are familiar with the area and have preselected locations to stop and use the restroom or to eat.

home visitors to resist hugging babies, changing diapers, helping with bottles, and so on. While some of these instrumental tasks can be helpful icebreakers, it can be risky, especially early in the relationship when you are unfamiliar with the home. Avoid this contact if possible. It is also wise to avoid touching pets. Another very difficult health-related issue has to do with accepting food and drink in the home. This is very difficult because there is often a cultural component to offering food. One option is to thank the family and tell them you will bring it back to the office or to your home to eat later.

THE VISIT

Every visit with a family, including the very first one, has a structure and a rhythm. Because many overburdened families need a sense of continuity, the more you can organize every contact so that it follows a similar flow, the more likely it is that the family will begin to trust in the process and feel they can count on you. In a very real way, the structure you provide is like a "holding environment"; this is a way of describing the comfort and security associated with knowing what to expect and having confidence that the relationship will remain stable, even though many things are changing for the family. From the very first visit, it is important to provide the family with the assurance, through your ability to structure the contact, that you are there for them.

Beginning

Once you and the family have settled down to begin your first interview, you will want to work on establishing rapport. Remember that rapport is based on trust. It is not realistic to think that just because you come from a program that offers help to families that they will automatically trust you. Trust has to be earned, and with families who have had difficult experiences in the past, it can be very fragile. While developing initial trust is vital to even engaging the family in a helping relationship, it would be wise for you to remind yourself before each and every visit that you need to earn and maintain the family's trust.

When you first meet the family, the first thing to do is to break the ice. You can begin this process by introducing yourself and acknowledging all family members who are present. Try to make eye contact and interact with each member of the family, even if it is only a brief interaction. Find out if there is anyone else whom the family thinks should be involved in the visits, and encourage the family to invite those individuals to subsequent meetings. Be tentative. Do not walk in as if the family is already prepared to get to work on issues of concern. Go slow. Take the time to show each family member that you are interested in him or her. At this ice-breaking stage it is important to be aware of cultural differences and expectations. Let the family know that you are interested in their point of view and that you are not going to force them to follow yours.

Introduce reciprocity through modeling. Many overburdened families are used to authoritarian relationships in which they are told what to do and do not own either the behaviors or the outcomes. Invite family members to lead, to tell you what they want, and what they think about their current situation. There is often a fine balance between responding to the family's urgent requests for advice, information, and even instructions, and helping them to take an active part in the articulation of their concerns and the solutions. Avoid the trap of being the "expert." Help the family to recognize that you think they are the experts in solving their problems. By providing a structured opportunity to reflect and plan, and by giving the family a chance to respond to a relationship that is consistent, you will be opening up an opportunity for them to actively control their world. Showing confidence right from the beginning will encourage trust.

It is difficult to avoid experiencing anxiety and sharing the family's sense of being overwhelmed. The sources of anxiety are many. For one thing the family may be involved in activities that frighten you such as substance abuse, crime, and family violence. For another, the process of referral,

---

SIDEBAR 3.4

Structure of the Initial Visit

I. Beginning
   A. Break the ice, establish rapport.
   B. Start "where the client is."
   C. Explain confidentiality.
II. Middle
   A. Discuss the referral, hopes, concerns.
   B. Use active listening, engagement, and communication skills.
   C. Assess functioning and current risk.
   D. Get "hired" by the family.
III. End
   A. Review and summarize the visit.
   B. Plan for the next contact.
   C. Agree upon any activities to take place in the interim.
   D. Encourage feedback/reflection about the visit.
IV. Follow through
   A. Document the visit.
   B. Review with your supervisor/team.
   C. Self-reflection and identification of concerns, possible countertransference,* and other areas in which you will need support.
   D. Develop some tentative ideas about the scope of your work with the family.
   E. Follow up on any referrals or other activities that you agreed to.

* Countertransference refers to the home visitor's reactions, sometimes not fully conscious, to family members. Some countertransference reactions stem from the home visitor's own personal history, while others may be induced by contact with the family member. It is important to identify and manage countertransference reactions through supervision and reflection. These sometimes powerful responses to family members, when they are consciously acknowledged and managed, can be quite helpful in understanding key issues with which family members are struggling. Unrecognized countertransference reactions can be counterproductive.

---

in many cases, has identified deficits and risks, and you may feel pressure to fix the identified problems. Sometimes the referral source will say something like: "This mother needs to work on self-esteem and child discipline issues." While this may be true, let's take a moment to deconstruct this statement. The statement is actually a form of code and may mean that the mother has serious issues arising from her own development. She may have developmental challenges in several spheres that are now compounded by life events and circumstances, such as poverty, single motherhood, low educational attainment, and poor relationships with men. She may not know very much about child development, but more important, she herself may never have experienced a nurturing environment, so even with instruction, she may not know how to discipline or nurture her children. Underlying all of this is an assumption of deficit. The referring agent has told you that he/she thinks this is an inadequate parent who needs to be changed, and he/she has told you what they think you should do. However, if you reframe this expectation, it is possible to think about things differently. Rather than responding to the deficits, it is possible to reframe things. For instance, the mother might, with support, welcome the opportunity to achieve more mature development, and perhaps, by understanding her own needs more self-reflectively, she will be better able to engage her children with empathy and genuineness. It is important for you to approach the situation openly and with acceptance. This does not mean condoning behavior you think is risky or in some other way problematic, but it does mean that you can meet the family members at the maturation level at which they are currently functioning and assist them with developing new skills.

A corollary to the willingness to address the family at the level of maturation and functioning with which it is operating is the need to allow them to stay where they are if they want to. As difficult as it is to accept, some families are not ready or willing to engage in a growth process. Client self-determination means that clients have the right not to engage in a relationship if they so choose. This may have consequences for an individual family, and the consequences may be significant. Families may become separated and people may go to jail. While these outcomes are the opposite of what family-support programs are all about, it is important that you recognize that the family and its members may choose these adverse outcomes over growth and it is not your job to force them to do otherwise. However, your job is to offer alternatives and to provide the level of support, the holding environment that will enable growth if the family so chooses. During the ice-breaking stage you may not know the family's intentions. In fact they may not be sure either. Most likely they are ambivalent and nervous about what might happen. If you present yourself as a caring, consistent person with good boundaries and with a sense of hope for the family, even those who are ambivalent may well give it a try.

Similarly, early in the conversation you will want to reassure the family about issues of confidentiality. The family needs to know that their confidentiality will be protected except in situations in which they or others might be placed in danger. You will need to tell them that you are required to report child abuse and that suicidal or violent behavior may result in police intervention. If the client has been mandated to participate you will want to talk through how information will be shared with the agency that has jurisdiction over their case. Most programs have a release of information form that allows clients to give permission to share information. Make sure you have release of information forms with you.

Your program may also use a "consent to services" form. If so, you will need to review it with the family and obtain their consent to enter the program. Ideally the consent to services form provides protection for family members by ensuring that they are giving informed consent to participate in the program. This means that family members need to be provided with information about what the program is, what activities you might be carrying out and why, risks they might incur, and potential benefits. Informed consent allows the family member to be a partner in the family-support process rather than a recipient. The difference may seem subtle, but it represents an important way to empower the family and to engage family members in taking responsibility and control for their participation in the family-support home-visiting case-management process.

We will talk more about issues of confidentiality in chapter 8. For now it is important for you to let the family know you are protecting their confidentiality and to give them as much control as possible over what information is shared with others.

Middle

Once you have completed mutual introductions and reviewed with the family what your program does, it is important to find out from them what they think they need or want from the relationship with you. Most families will not have a clear picture of what they want, so it will be important to carefully tease out their experiences, their current understanding of what is happening, and their hopes for the future. You will need to use active listening and communications skills in order to help the family articulate their hopes and expectations. In the middle part of the interview, you might ask the family a form of what practitioners of solution-focused intervention call the "Miracle Question" (DeJong and Berg 2002): "If you woke up tomorrow and everything was the way it should be, what would it look like? What would be happening? What would be different?" This is important because right from the beginning the family begins to develop a vision and a sense of the future.

In the middle phase of the interview you will also be doing an initial assessment of risk and current functioning. In chapter 5 we will explore more about risk assessment. You will want to determine, at least on a preliminary level, how the family is doing and if immediate intervention is required.

Perhaps the most important part of the interview is a discussion with the family about whether they want to participate in the program, and specifically, whether they want to engage in a working relationship with you. One way to think about this is that the family is "hiring" you to help facilitate their growth and development. Do not assume that just because you are in the home for this first visit that they want to continue. Try to have an open, honest discussion with them about their expectations, concerns, and needs and about whether or not they see working with you as a means to address things that concern them.

SIDEBAR 3.5

Empowering Communications Skills

Respect/acceptance: This is reflected in body language, facial expressions, and demeanor that is nonjudgmental and communicates to the client that you are interested and that they can "tell you anything" without fear that you will judge or criticize them.

Empathic listening: Using techniques such as open-ended questions, paraphrasing, reflection of content, and feelings reflects this. You convey to the client that you are paying attention and understand what he/she is telling you.

Following: This is a special instance of empathic listening in which the helper stays close to the content being expressed by the client. Identifying latent emotional content and using paraphrasing, reframing, questions, and reflection help you to keep pace with the client's thoughts and feelings. Be specific: "I notice you are responding very honestly to Janet when she asks where her daddy is."

Normalizing: Help the family to recognize that they are not alone in their experiences. Reframe self-criticisms and feelings of being different so the family member can see that their experiences can be understood in a nonpathological way. This increases the family's internal solidarity and encourages family members to reduce isolation and join with others who may have similar concerns.

Tentative attitude: Try to avoid "telling" the family, and present your ideas in a way that allows the family to back away if they are not ready to see things your way. Wondering, asking for feedback on ideas, and being careful not to present yourself as a "know-it-all" will help the family feel open to explore and experiment. Use "wondering" as a way to enable the client to reject an idea without being afraid you will feel personally rejected. "I'm wondering if it would help to set his alarm five or ten minutes earlier so he won't be late."

Focus and structure: Without being rigid, follow a structure and help keep the conversation focused. When the client starts to wander or to become repetitive, in a tentative, respectful way, return to the structure. "Would it be okay with you if we reviewed what we have talked about so far, and maybe think about what you would like to do about talking to Sandy's teacher?"

Cultural awareness and competence: It is important to families that they be allowed to integrate new ideas and behaviors into existing cultural and value paradigms. You will need to be familiar with meanings from the client's perspective, and culture is a key component of understanding what things mean to a family member.

Accept, articulate, and contain strong emotions: Clients need to feel free to express their feelings. You may find it necessary to help them articulate their feelings and tease out more specific meanings. For instance, "I feel bad" may need to be clarified and teased out. Does "bad" mean angry, sad, sick, guilty, ashamed, or something else? It is vital that no matter how strong the emotion, or how unpleasant, the client knows that you will not avoid the emotion, criticize them, or try to talk them out of what they are feeling. Allowing emotions to be put into words often reduces their power.

If the family members are ambivalent, do not push for closure, but rather, ask them how they would like to proceed. They may need to think about it, or contact the referring agency or individual. Family members may be reluctant and will appreciate your acceptance of this reaction. Even if they decide not to continue at this time, if the experience of deciding can be as empowering as possible, it will be easier for the family to seek help in the future. In the next chapter we will talk more about assessing motivation and readiness to change. If the family is not ready to commit, move to the ending part of the interview gracefully, without making the family feel they have failed or hurt your feelings. "So, Mrs. James, right now it seems like you are not sure that all of this is really necessary. I understand your feelings. It is a big decision, and you are right to be careful about it. Why don't we summarize and end for now, and I'll leave you my card."

Ending the Interview

At the end of the interview, you should

1. Review and summarize today's visit.
2. Plan for the next meeting. If the family has not committed to participate, make sure that they have the information they will need to contact you if they decide later that they want to engage in a relationship.
3. Agree on next steps: "I will come by next Monday at 3 P.M." "You have my card. If you decide to participate in the program, call me."
4. Encourage the client to provide feedback and reflection on the session. Are there any things they are concerned about? Do they have questions?

As you leave the home, make sure to thank the family for their time and for inviting you into their home.

Follow Through

Once the visit is over, you will want to document what happened. Most agencies use progress notes or ask home visitors to make notes on the referral form to indicate whether the family will be opened in the program. Make a note of questions or issues you will need to review with your supervisor or team. Think about your reactions to the interview and to the family. It is important to engage in honest self-reflection and to identify any countertransference issues, judgments, or anxieties that you have. Countertransference usually refers to the reactions and feelings, often unconscious, of the helper. Many times, if there is a countertransference reaction, the home visitor will find himself or herself having atypical reactions to a particular client. You may feel like bringing a family member home with you to take care of them, or you may be irrationally angry with a family for letting you down in some way. The home visitor may find himself or herself making excuses for the family or being unusually impatient with them. These reactions may come from the home visitor's own history or developmental challenges, or the family may induce them. Emotional reactions emerging from the home visitor's own history are sources of subjective countertransference (Spotnitz 1995), and may be a source of counterproductive activities and exchanges in the relationship with the family. Induced countertransference (Spotnitz 1995), on the other hand, refers to feelings that most people might have in response to the family. These reactions may well be responses to subtle communication of needs and challenges by the family. It is important to be honest with yourself and engage in frank self-reflection when you find that you are having strong reactions to a family, especially if those reactions lead you to contemplate actions that are inconsistent with your normal approach or with the boundaries set by program policies and your own training. Be sure to discuss these concerns with your supervisor and your team. By articulating your questions and concerns you will be able to look at them more objectively and identify action steps to resolve them.

You should also be formulating a preliminary assessment of risk, functioning, goals, and thinking through a potential action plan. Make sure that you follow up on any referrals or activities you told the family you would carry out. The family will learn to trust you and have confidence in you if you follow through with commitments. The reverse is also true. If you disappoint them or do not do what you have said you would do, the family will have evidence that you are not trustworthy and that they cannot count on you. Overburdened families frequently feel that others are not trustworthy and that they cannot count on people, so failure to follow through can be potentially destructive in that you are further convincing the family members that there is little hope for them. Of course, there are times that you agree to do something, and even though you try, it cannot be accomplished. Going back to the family and letting them know what happened will let them know that you did follow through, but that another way to accomplish the task will need to be identified. In this case the family may put you on "probation," thinking that you are well meaning and honest, but ineffective. It is important to tease these feelings out and to stay with the family as they express disappointment and together you seek alternatives. This will help them see that you do keep your word and that you will not abandon them even if things become a little difficult. The key here is your commitment to doing what you say and being able to demonstrate to the family you are still with them, even if your effort was not initially successful.

Resist the temptation to fix everything or to jump into action, but instead focus on trying to understand the family, the perspectives of its members, and some of the things that might be helpful to them. It is too early to lock yourself into a course of action, but you should be reviewing and evaluating possibilities. Your supervisor and team will probably have some good ideas about what is going on, and some action steps that might be useful. At this stage you are collecting information and formulating hypotheses. This can be a little disconcerting because it will feel like you should do something right now. However, the most important thing you can do is to continue the assessment until you and the family are really clear about what is going on, what their goals are, and if and how you can help.

SUMMARY

This chapter explores the first stage of working with a family. It is important to engage the family and to be aware of the fragile nature of the relationship in its early stages.

SIDEBAR 3.6

The Rodriguez Family

The Family-Support Case-Management Program

Parenting for Healthy Children is a comprehensive family-support program that is part of a large, well-established community agency whose mission it is to provide a broad array of health, mental health, and social services in the community of Gatewood, a blighted area of a large city. The program has the following goals:

1. Preventing child abuse and neglect
2. Enhancing school readiness
3. Promoting positive parenting skills
4. Promoting the health and well-being of family members
5. Preventing adverse outcomes for children and families
6. Promoting family self-sufficiency

To accomplish these goals, the Parenting for Health program provides a wide array of services, including

1. Parenting classes
2. Life skills classes
3. Child development groups
4. Psychotherapy
5. Case management
   a. Home visitors
   b. Linkage to primary health care
   c. Linkage to substance abuse and mental health treatment

The program has been funded to work with families identified to be at risk by the local pediatric hospital. Families are identified during the first year of the child's life and referred to the program. Services are offered on a voluntary basis for a period of three years.

A team consisting of a social worker, a nurse, a child development specialist, a substance abuse specialist, a parent educator, and five home visitors provides services. Either a nurse or a master's level social worker manages each team. Each team works with 100–125 families, providing case-management and family-support services.

The Family

Enrique and Sofia Rodriguez and their eight-month-old son, Omar, were referred by the nurse in the pediatric clinic to the Parenting for Health program after Omar was diagnosed for the third time with impetigo. The nurse indicated that the couple did not seem to understand how to prevent these infections and how to maintain hygiene in the home. She also indicated that the baby did not seem to be developing normally and appeared not to be securely attached to either parent. The parents spoke English, although Enrique seemed to be more comfortable speaking Spanish. The nurse felt that the case manager for the family should probably be fluent in Spanish. The nurse agreed to send along the family's release of information permission and other basic demographic information

Initial Engagement

The team leader assigned the family to Linda, a Spanish-speaking home visitor with several years of experience in family-support case management. In reading the information provided by the referring nurse, Linda learned that Enrique is a twenty-nine-year-old laborer, who works for several landscaping companies. He has no health insurance for the family. Sofia is twenty-four years old. She dropped out of high school when she was fifteen years old and began cleaning homes. She has tried off and on to return to this work since Omar was born, but has no childcare and most of her steady patrons have made other arrangements. The family lives in a one-bedroom apartment. The referral information indicates that Omar was a low birth weight baby and that he has continued to be on the low end of height, weight, and developmental charts. There does not seem to be family nearby. Sofia's family is in another city in the United States, and Enrique's family lives in Mexico in a border city.

(Continued next page)

Linda tried several times to reach the family by telephone, but received a busy signal each time. Finally, while out in the field on another visit, Linda dropped a note in the door of the Rodriguez apartment, indicating a day and time that she would try to meet the family.

When Linda arrived, a slightly overweight, disheveled young woman greeted her. A baby was sitting in a walker. The baby wore a t-shirt and was barefoot. There was dried milk on his face and an empty bottle nearby on the floor. There were no toys. The television was on at a high volume. The young woman did not make eye contact and was distracted, looking from the home visitor to her television show. After a few uncomfortable silences, the young woman finally blurted out, "Why are you here?" Linda indicated that she had been asked by the nurse at the pediatrician's office to meet Sofia and see if any of the services of the Parenting for Healthy Children program would be of any interest to her. Sofia was skeptical, but wondered if the program offered free diapers and childcare. Linda talked a little bit about the program and offered to leave the program brochure with Sofia, who was noncommittal. Sofia was hesitant to make a second appointment, and told Linda she would call the agency if she were interested.

Linda reviewed the visit with her team and indicated that she was concerned about the condition of the home, Sofia's emotional distance, and the status of the baby. The team recognized that there were possibly attachment issues, and perhaps some depression in Sofia, but recognized that since the case is voluntary, the best that could be done would be some additional nonintrusive outreach, with the hope that Sofia would be willing at a later time to engage in a relationship with the home visitor.

Several weeks later, Sofia called Linda and indicated that she was not interested in the program, but would like to get some information about childcare. She gave Linda permission to come to her apartment to drop off some information. Linda stopped by Sofia's apartment on the way to another home visit. They chatted for a few moments, and Linda left, making sure that Sofia knew that she could contact her again. Over the next few weeks, Sofia called for small things, such as information about WIC, questions about GED programs in the community, and the schedule of the parenting classes offered by the program. Linda suggested that if Sofia attended a class that perhaps they could meet for a few minutes afterwards to "debrief." Sofia indicated that she could not really come to class because she had no way to get there and did not know what to do with Omar. Linda talked to her about the childcare available through the program for parents attending the groups, and provided details about what to bring for Omar, and how things would work. Since the program offered taxi vouchers for parents just starting in the parenting groups, Linda offered to drop a round trip voucher off at the apartment. When Linda arrived with the voucher, Sofia stood at the door asking many questions about the details of when to feed Omar, when to bring him. She also had many questions about what the group would be like and what to expect. Linda patiently answered all of the questions, and Sofia said she felt fairly comfortable about attending the class.

Sofia attended her first class and spoke briefly with Linda after the class. After coming to two classes, Sofia arrived with Enrique. After the class both Enrique and Sofia spent some time in Linda's office, asking questions about the program and about child development. During the conversation Linda told the couple a little about family support and asked if they would like to try it. Both Enrique and Sofia indicate that they think it might help them solve some of their day-to-day financial problems, and made an appointment with Linda for the following Wednesday.

It is noteworthy that Linda did not "push" the family, but remained open, nonjudgmental and matter-of-fact. As the family became more familiar with Linda and the program and more comfortable with their interactions with program staff, they were more open to the idea of engaging in the program. At this point the family has "hired" Linda to work with them.

Preparation for the initial contact, along with some suggestions for structuring the first contact is presented. The home visitor is encouraged to utilize supervision and other team members to carefully reflect upon their initial reactions to families. Suggestions for organizing the information obtained in the initial contact and for maintaining momentum are offered.

FOUR

Systematic Assessment

In the last chapter we examined some of the ways that families are selected to partici-pate in family-support programs. Some programs are voluntary and can be universally offered or selectively offered, based on specific risk factors. Other programs, such as child protective services or programs ordered by the courts are mandated, and are often risk based. Regardless of the method used to identify families, once they enter the program a systematic assessment of functioning on several dimensions must take place in order to provide the kind of support families need to improve their day-to-day coping skills.

Figure 4.1 Systematic assessment

Family-Support Home-Visiting Case-Management Process

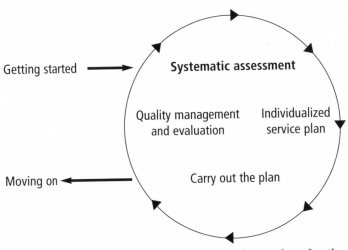

Systematic assessment is a vital part of providing family-support home-visiting case management, since it provides you and the family with guidance about where to start, and what to do as you carry out your work together. Assessment is both a *process* and a *product* (Hepworth 2006). This means that as a process, assessment is something that you DO, an activity that you carry out, and at the same time, the process results in an assessment summary that presents your best understanding of the current situation. The assessment process is ongoing, and the resulting understanding evolves as you obtain more information about the family and the context in which its members are functioning. The process of assessment involves gathering as much information as possible from various sources, and then organizing and reorganizing the information as you and the family gain deeper understanding of the situation. The process begins as soon as you receive the referral and continues right up to the last visit with the family. At the end of your work with a family, both you and they should have a good idea about what brought them to request services, what the needs are and have been, what history and precursors affected the issues confronting the family, and what resources and specific interventions were helpful in resolving the issues. The process of assessment will help identify what is needed and how things are going at each step of the family-support home-visiting process.

Every time that you meet with the family, you should be looking at how they are doing, changes in any risk factors, as well as any changes in family members' motivation or commitment to the process of change. Essentially the process of assessment helps you to stay in touch with what is going on with the family and to adjust what you do based on changes or new information. It is very important to keep the assessment process open and ongoing in order to assure that what you do continues to be relevant to the family. This means that even after a product (the assessment report or summary) has been prepared, your assessment task is not over. Simply completing an assessment report and filing it as one more completed task to tick off your list is not enough; the assessment process needs to continue in every contact with the family.

You may very well be wondering what it is that should be included in an assessment. It is best to start by thinking about what you are doing and why. You are collecting information on a number of dimensions in order to get a good understanding of the person in his or her environment. You will use this information to help develop goals and an intervention plan. A good assessment is key to identifying the family's needs, capacities, commitment to change, and goals. Family-support case management looks at the individual and family within his/her social, cultural, and community context. Figure 4.2 illustrates this point.

A multidimensional assessment involves looking at both strengths and challenges at the individual, family, community, and social levels. While the home visitor may only be targeting the individual or family level, it is important to understand how community and social factors serve as protective or vulnerability factors. Protective factors are those elements of the situation that help enhance functioning or work to reduce the effects of factors that may be adverse or risk producing. Conversely risk factors are those elements that contribute to barriers, challenges, and adverse outcomes. These concepts from resiliency theory (Rutter 1987; Garbarino 1995; Davies 1999; Shonkoff and Phillips 2000) are important to keep in mind when doing an assessment. You will be looking for factors, either in the person, his/her support systems, or environmental context that either promote or inhibit optimal functioning and well-being. Identifying a vulnerability factor is not a criticism, nor should it lead to a sense of hopelessness. Instead, you should try to find all of the things in a situation that move the family in a positive direction, and then identify those elements of the situation that

Figure 4.2　Understanding the person-in-environment

Social and political context

Environment

Economy

Communities

Group and organizations

Reciprocal interactions:
Protective factors
Vulnerability (risk) factors

Family

Culture

Individual

Social Class

Genetics and health

History

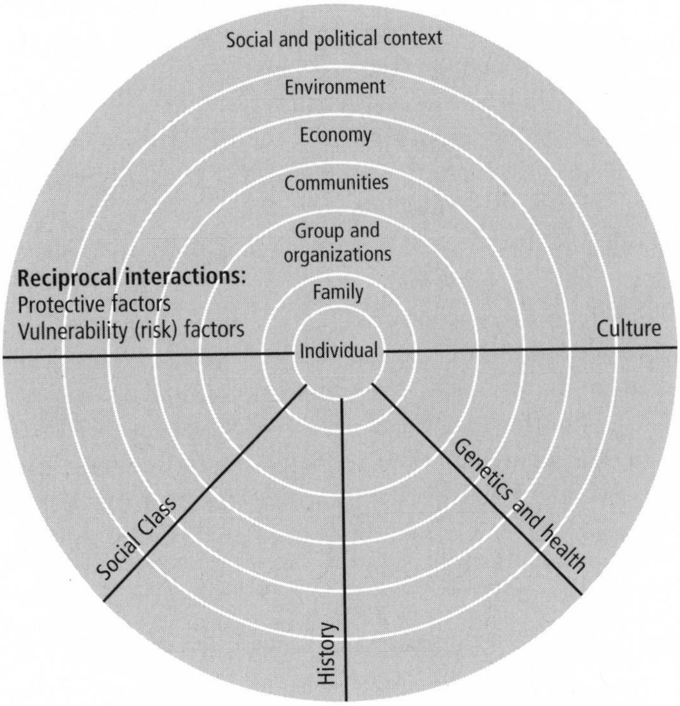

SIDEBAR 4.1

Assessment Reminders

Remember:

- An assessment is nothing more than the compilation of information from different places. It is not "written in stone" and changes as new information deepens your understanding.
- An assessment is not a diagnosis; it is more like a working hypothesis about what is going on.
- You may use diagnostic information, psychological test information, and standardized test information to help you understand things, but none of these tools by itself provides a complete picture of the person-in-environment constellation.
- A realistic assessment of things is different than a criticism of the individual or family. It simply allows you and the family to note things that are relevant and important as you set your goals and plan your work together.

need to be overcome, removed, changed, or otherwise addressed in order to enhance well-being.

It should be clear from the discussion so far that the process of assessment is complex and dynamic. You will need to always keep in mind the balance between vulnerability and protective factors. You are probably wondering where the information for an assessment comes from, and what information you should be collecting. Sidebars 4.2 and 4.3 summarize some key information that you will want to explore during the assessment process.

ASSESSING CURRENT RISK

Overburdened families may evidence high-risk behaviors that present concerns for the safety of family members, yourself, or others in the community. It is important to be

1. From the initial referral materials. Things like the intake form, the initial referral, and even service and assessment summaries from the referral source provide important background information.

2. From the client. The individual family member or family as a whole will give you information about what they see as the problems and concerns facing them.

3. Your own observations of how the family members present themselves and how they interact with you, with each other, and other people will provide you with important information.

4. Information from other people who have contact with the family provides insight. Some of these individuals can include, among others, teachers, lawyers, counselors, professionals at other agencies, clergy, and other staff in your program who have had contact with the family.

5. Standardized tests and assessment tools

I. Current risks
  A. Violence Potential (including suicide and homicide)
  B. Substance use/abuse
  C. Family violence
    1. Child abuse and neglect
    2. Partner/domestic violence
    3. Elder abuse
  D. Mental health concerns
  E. Traumatic loss/crisis

II. Developmental considerations and past history
  A. Psychosocial/developmental status of individual family members
  B. Individual and family biography and history/unresolved issues
  C. Individual and family life cycle stages
  D. Health/medical history
  E. Personal and cultural expectations

III. Current functioning
  A. Living situation
  B. Adequacy of role functioning
  C. Stresses
  D. Educational/vocational circumstances
  E. Quality of relationships
  F. Coping and adaptive skills of family members
  G. Family dynamics

IV. Social and environmental factors
  A. Neighborhood resources/barriers
  B. Legal issues, criminal involvement
  C. Race, ethnicity, culture
  D. Class
  E. Gender
  F. Cultural affiliations
  G. Social and environmental factors

V. Readiness to change

realistic and aware of risks, while at the same time avoiding overreacting or distancing from the family. Treating the risks matter of factly, without criticism, and without condoning high-risk behavior requires training and support. Most home-visiting programs provide training in domestic violence, child abuse, substance abuse, suicide risk, and mental health. Consult your supervisor regularly to help understand high-risk situations. At the beginning of every home visit you should get in the habit of doing a mini assessment to identify any changes in risk level since your last visit. Plan in advance how you will handle these changes. The key to effective family-support case management is continuity and steadiness; the home visitor will need to identify changes in risk and potential crises. While not every crisis can be averted, careful attention to the here-and-now risks will help assure stability and safety for you and the family.

MANAGING CRISIS SITUATIONS

It is not always possible to avoid crisis situations. A crisis is a sudden, often unexpected, overwhelming situation that breaks the normal flow of things. Many of the families requiring family-support services experience multiple and frequent crises. One of the things that you can do to help is to sort out what is happening with the family and help them to recognize the difference between an unpleasant or anxiety-provoking situation and a true crisis. What is experienced as a crisis can differ dramatically from

■

SIDEBAR 4.4

Risk Factor Checklist

Consider the items below and determine the family's level of risk on each factor. You may want to assess each family member separately.

Score	Risk Factor				
___	1. **Suicide**	5 high risk	4 considerable risk	3 moderate risk	2 slight risk	1 no risk/low risk
___	2. **Violent behavior**	5 high risk	4 considerable risk	3 moderate risk	2 slight risk	1 no risk/low risk
___	3. **Depression**	5 high risk	4 considerable risk	3 moderate risk	2 slight risk	1 no risk/low risk
___	4. **Psychosis**	5 high risk	4 considerable risk	3 moderate risk	2 slight risk	1 no risk/low risk
___	5. **Anxiety**	5 high risk	4 considerable risk	3 moderate risk	2 slight risk	1 no risk/low risk
___	6. **Alcohol abuse**	5 high risk	4 considerable risk	3 moderate risk	2 slight risk	1 no risk/low risk
___	7. **Drug abuse**	5 high risk	4 considerable risk	3 moderate risk	2 slight risk	1 no risk/low risk
___	8. **Domestic violence**	5 high risk	4 considerable risk	3 moderate risk	2 slight risk	1 no risk/low risk
___	9. **Child abuse**	5 high risk	4 considerable risk	3 moderate risk	2 slight risk	1 no risk/low risk
___	10. **Elder abuse**	5 high risk	4 considerable risk	3 moderate risk	2 slight risk	1 no risk/low risk
___	11. **Overall risk**	5 high risk	4 considerable risk	3 moderate risk	2 slight risk	1 no risk/low risk

Developed by Terry Carrilio and Sally Mathieson, San Diego State University person to person. Often it is not the actual situation, but the perception of, and reaction to, the situation *at this time*. It is important to remember the protective/vulnerability concept that we discussed with respect to resiliency. What this means is that at different times people are more or less vulnerable to stress. If a family has had an accumulation of small problems, it may be that something fairly minor, such as a leaky roof, will push one or more members into a crisis, whereas, at another time, while the leaky roof would be an annoyance, it would not result in a crisis.

It is easy to see how major events, such as acts of nature, accidents, and other sudden traumas might result in a crisis experience. However, it is also important to recognize the "quiet crisis," which is sometimes harder to predict. Any transition, such as going to a new school, finishing an important task, such as graduating from high school, experiencing a life cycle event, such as giving birth, getting married, and acclimating to an "empty nest, "depending on the balance of risk and vulnerability, and the meaning of the experience for the individual, can lead to a crisis experience. It is important to recognize that while life transitions may pose a source of vulnerability, this is not *necessarily* the case, and certainly does not mean that every transition in life must be crisis laden. However, it does mean that you should pay attention to transitions, even those that seem fairly mundane. If you do find yourself working with a family in crisis, you may wish to utilize some of the suggestions in sidebar 4.6.

SIDEBAR 4.5

Recognizing a Crisis

- Family members are overwhelmed and report being flooded with emotions and thoughts about the situation.
- Often the individual or family can identify the "straw that broke the camel's back." Crisis can be caused by an overwhelming event (for example, a fire, earthquake, tsunami, sudden accident, change in health status) or by an accumulation of seemingly minor events.
- The individual tries to respond, often repetitively, with his/her normal coping strategies. When these normal ways of coping with stress fail, the individual feels out of control and unable to respond.
- The individual reports feeling helpless, angry, and out of control. There will be preoccupation with the situation of concern and often a focus on one or more concrete details of the situation.
- Various tactics to cope with the tension will be tried, often repetitively. Some of these tactics may represent regressions to earlier developmental levels and may be adaptive or maladaptive.
- The individual reports active discomfort and is often desperate to find solutions to relieve the tension and discomfort.
- The experience of being overwhelmed and out of control is recent and has not been going on for more than eight weeks.

ASSESSING DEVELOPMENTAL ISSUES AND PAST HISTORY

It will be important for you to have a basic understanding of family members' developmental history and current life cycle issues. While you will not be providing in-depth counseling as part of family-support case management, you will want to be aware of the way past traumas, health problems, unresolved traumas, and relationship problems might affect what is going on today and how family members respond to

---

SIDEBAR 4.6

Crisis Intervention Tips

You will be assessing the situation and reducing distress at the same time.

- What you will assess:
  - Level of risk (suicide, violence, psychotic episode, and so on)
  - Amount of discomfort and tension experienced by the individual
  - Adaptive capacities
  - Current and previous levels of functioning
  - Current level of distress and potential to act upon it
  - Recent life events (traumas, transitions, identified stresses)
- Focus on problems of living right now rather than on pathology—keep a "here and now" focus.
- Develop a crisis plan. Work with the family to clearly and specifically articulate what needs to happen and who will do it. Check in frequently and change the plan as new developments indicate.
- Recognize that a crisis is time limited (four to six weeks). The outcome is not certain; the family may be doing much better at the end of the crisis, having used the opportunity to develop new coping mechanisms, or the family may be doing much worse, utilizing problem solving and coping skills that are less effective than in the past.
- Maintain boundaries and try to avoid doing things for the family. This will increase their sense of being able to control things. Encourage family members to participate actively in developing and implementing the crisis plan.

---

current issues. You will want to learn a little bit about any mental health or substance abuse history. It will be important to look at how family members have functioned in various roles, such as student, employee, parent, spouse, sibling, and friend.

As you learn about the family's past history and developmental challenges that have faced each family member, it is important to pay attention not only to what actually happened, but also to the family member's *experience* of what happened. Cultural and gender expectations will need to be explored. It is important to understand how the family understands their own history and development, and whether they feel that this development is congruent with their expectations. Try to elicit information about what happened as well as what the family members thought and felt about what happened. This will help you to develop an understanding of areas of sensitivity, concern, and pride for family members. As you work with the family, this understanding can help you and the family to better understand instances in which family members seem stuck, or experience unexpected emotional reactions to events.

One way to learn a bit more about family members is to follow up on statements they make. Here are some examples:

Parent: Joe is a terrible child. He acts just like his !@#$%! father.

Home visitor: It sounds like this concerns you. What kinds of things did his dad do that you are concerned about?

Parent: I don't want to end up like my sister, living on welfare and being depressed all the time.

Home visitor: I wonder if you can tell me a little bit about your ideas of how your sister got that way?

This kind of background information can tell you something about events that are meaningful to the parent, and how these past events might affect current behaviors.

Assessing Current Functioning

It is important to find out how the family and its individual members are doing on a day-to-day basis. The assessment of current functioning is something that you should do quickly every time you meet with the family.

In most cases you will be recording your own impressions, and sometimes the family's impressions, of how they are doing in these areas. Once you have a general picture of how the family is doing, you, your supervisor, and the family will be better able to identify goals for your work together. In addition to the items described in the checklist in sidebar 4.7, you will want to obtain a picture of the family's current living circumstances. It is important to understand the composition of the household and to clarify the way that relationships between household members may reduce or enhance current stresses.

Assessing Social and Environmental Factors

An assessment of the social environment includes things like housing, transportation, and the ready availability of resources such as shopping, schools, and places of worship. It is important to look at how organized the neighborhood and larger community are and how resources can be used to support the family. The larger social context may also present barriers that need to be addressed. Lack of needed resources, lack of community safety, violence, housing concerns, and transportation can present serious barriers to families. It is important to identify people and institutions in the community that might be helpful to the family. A useful tool in organizing your observations about the social and environmental context is the ecomap (McPhatter 1991). This tool puts the dynamic situation of the family into a graphic format that is sometimes quite revealing. If possible, the home visitor should involve the family in the creation of the ecomap. Frequently family members find this both enlightening and empowering. Sometimes just seeing the situation in a simple, graphic form helps the family to see what needs to change. This tool also gives the home visitor an excellent way to present the concepts of strengths and barriers in a way that makes sense to the family.

The family's religious, racial, ethnic, and cultural background should be part of the assessment of social and environmental factors. It is helpful to know how involved the family is with cultural and religious institutions, and whether these relationships are supportive or conflictual. In situations in which language, culture, ethnicity, race, religion, or gender are important to the family's identity and social resources, it is sometimes helpful to do a culturagram (Congress 1994). This is a way of looking at the relative effects of the family's primary identifications. For some families, ethnic, racial, religious, and cultural considerations are in the forefront. For others it is important information, but not central in the family's worldview.

Figure 4.3 Social and community context: the ecomap

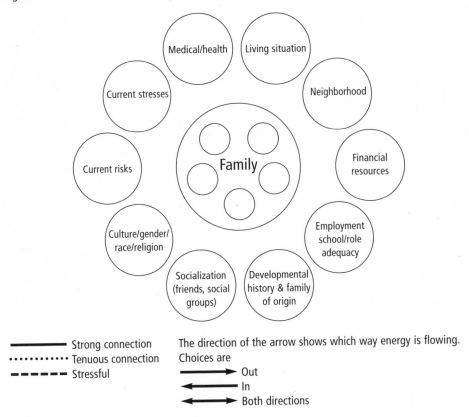

Strong connection
Tenuous connection
Stressful

The direction of the arrow shows which way energy is flowing.
Choices are

Out
In
Both directions

Try to address each of these areas with the family. Write notes on the bottom and the back of the diagram to explain things. Try to determine whether each dimension is supportive or stressful. Use this diagram to get a quick snapshot of some of the key strengths and challenges facing the family. Depending on the complexity of the situation and the scope of your program's work with the family, you might want to do an ecomap for each individual family member. Remember, this is a guide and will change as the family's circumstances change.

■

SIDEBAR 4.7

Current Functioning Checklist

1. Start with how the individual or family is doing with respect to carrying out key activities of daily life.

Area of functioning	Level of functioning				
Relationships with family	1 Very low	2 Poor	3 Adequate	4 Good	5 Excellent
Relationships in the community	1 Very low	2 Poor	3 Adequate	4 Good	5 Excellent
School/work	1 Very low	2 Poor	3 Adequate	4 Good	5 Excellent
Adequacy of role functioning	1 Very low	2 Poor	3 Adequate	4 Good	5 Excellent
Coping and adaptive skills	1 Very low	2 Poor	3 Adequate	4 Good	5 Excellent
Health	1 Very low	2 Poor	3 Adequate	4 Good	5 Excellent
Self-care	1 Very low	2 Poor	3 Adequate	4 Good	5 Excellent
Parenting	1 Very low	2 Poor	3 Adequate	4 Good	5 Excellent

2. Now look at the severity of current stressors in the family's life.

Area of functioning	Level of problems				
Relationships with family	1 Significant	2 Noticeable	3 Moderate	4 Mild	5 None
Relationships in the community	1 Significant	2 Noticeable	3 Moderate	4 Mild	5 None
School/work	1 Significant	2 Noticeable	3 Moderate	4 Mild	5 None
Adequacy of role functioning	1 Significant	2 Noticeable	3 Moderate	4 Mild	5 None
Coping and adaptive skills	1 Significant	2 Noticeable	3 Moderate	4 Mild	5 None
Health	1 Significant	2 Noticeable	3 Moderate	4 Mild	5 None
Self-care	1 Significant	2 Noticeable	3 Moderate	4 Mild	5 None
Parenting	1 Significant	2 Noticeable	3 Moderate	4 Mild	5 None
Other	1 Significant	2 Noticeable	3 Moderate	4 Mild	5 None

Figure 4.4 A simple culturagram

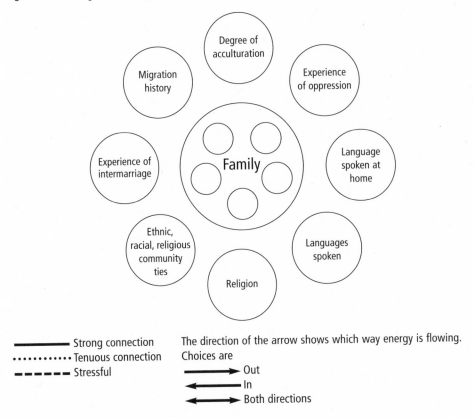

——————— Strong connection
•••••••••••• Tenuous connection
– – – – – Stressful

The direction of the arrow shows which way energy is flowing.
Choices are
———————▶ Out
◀——————— In
◀———————▶ Both directions

Try to address each of these areas with the family. Write notes on the bottom and the back of the diagram to explain things. Try to determine whether each dimension is supportive or stressful. Use this diagram to get a quick snapshot of some of the key strengths and challenges facing the family. Depending on the complexity of the situation and the scope of your program's work with the family, you might want to do an ecomap for each individual family member. Remember, this is a guide and will change as the family's circumstances change.

ASSESSING READINESS TO CHANGE

Many home visitors are confused when they find that the families they try to engage in the family-support case-management process are reluctant or disinterested. It is sometimes hard to understand how it is that even when people look like they are in pain, they would rather maintain the status quo than go through the challenge of change. Change is frightening because it involves the temporary disruption of established patterns and ways of doing things. Even when those patterns cause discomfort, they are familiar. It is important for the home visitor to recognize and appreciate that it takes courage to embark on any change. Just think of a time when you decided to change a habit. New Year's resolutions are a good example. We often make solemn promises to improve ourselves by exercising, eating better, gossiping less, or some other relatively small behavioral change. Most of us find excuses for continuing our overeating, talking too much, or whatever it is we were hoping to change. If we look a little deeper into what happened to those New Year's resolutions, what emerges is often that the new behavior is too much work, and the old one is comfortable and fits in with our overall way of ordering the world. Even if we are annoyed with ourselves for eating poorly, driving too fast, or engaging in other negative behaviors, most people drop New Year's resolutions because there is insufficient motivation to change, or the discomfort of the changes overwhelms the good intentions with which we started.

Change, even when it is something positive, can be disruptive. Naomi Golan addresses this when she talks about the process of transitions (1981). Systems theory also addresses this in the sense that the person or family as a system tries very hard to maintain a balance, a steady state, called homeostasis. The introduction of changes disrupts the homeostasis and puts the system into a position of vulnerability and uncertainty. All change involves risk. The home visitor's task is to provide a stable "holding environment" (Applegate and Bonnovitz 1995) for the family and its members as they transition from one steady state to another. Figure 4.5 illustrates the process of

Figure 4.5 The process of change: change is hard

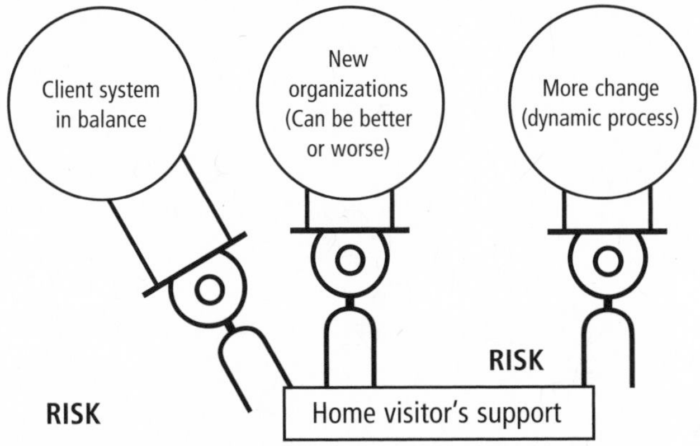

Developed by Terry Carrilio in collaboration with Mary Claire Heffron and Donna Weston, Social Policy Institute at San Diego State University

change as moving from one state of stable organization to another. In making the leap, there is always the risk of falling. The role of the home visitor is to help the family "make the leap" safely.

Clearly we are asking families to commit themselves to a difficult and sometimes frightening course of action. Let the family know that you are aware of how hard it is to commit to change. Make sure the family does not feel that they need to pretend they are interested in changing things just to please you or just to satisfy an external demand. Even when people *want* to change, it is difficult because they may not have a picture of what change looks like. One interesting approach to the need for a vision of something better is the "miracle question" (DeJong and Berg 2000). It involves asking the family, individually and collectively, what things would look like if miraculously the current problems disappeared. Asking the miracle question introduces the idea of hope and helps the family develop a vision to work toward. During the assessment, the family's responses to the miracle question give you information about what they would like for themselves as well as how strongly motivated they are to achieve these goals.

The stages of change model can be helpful in understanding both the different steps one passes through in the change process, and the process itself. This model suggests a five-stage change process that includes precontemplation, contemplation, preparation, action, and maintenance (Prochaska, DiClemente, and Norcross 1992). Utilizing this model, the home visitor assesses where the family is situated with respect to it readiness for change. If a family is in the early stages of recognizing the need to change things, it is important not to push too hard or to assume that just because the family is under external pressure to change they are ready to change. Jumping prematurely into interventions and action without assessing the family's readiness may lead to a premature end to the relationship. It is important to provide support and recognize that families in the early stages of thinking about change may not be ready at this time to engage in a relationship with the home visitor. By acknowledging this and helping the family to be honest about their level of commitment to the change process, you can prevent frustration for both parties. Remember: If the family is at an early stage of readiness to change, the way that you handle things may influence their willingness to seek help at a later time.

USING STANDARDIZED ASSESSMENT TOOLS

Your program may ask you to fill out standardized assessment forms to help identify key concerns of families. A standardized assessment is a set of questions or structured observations that have been empirically tested, and have been shown to provide valid and reliable information. Usually the information reflects one of the dimensions above, such as depression, suicide risk, child abuse potential, or dimensions of functioning. Sometimes a standardized instrument will look at attitudes or personal characteristics. A standardized instrument has been tested on different groups of people. Often programs will choose to use standardized assessments that have been previously tested on populations similar to the clients they serve. These standardized measures can be very helpful in identifying areas of concern that might not be immediately obvious, such as underlying depression or mental health concerns. They can also be very helpful, as we will discuss later, in helping you to track progress over time. If your program asks you to use one or more standardized assessment tools, think of them as tools to help you understand the family. Use of standardized instruments is strongly encouraged, since these measures provide the home visitor and team leader with an idea of how the family is doing relative to a larger population, and permit pre and post-comparisons of how the family has done while in the program.

WRITING UP THE ASSESSMENT

Sometimes it is helpful to use a structured worksheet to help you organize your observations. Sidebar 4.8 gives an example of an assessment summary. You might want to adapt something like this to help you and the family understand the current situation and some of the dynamics affecting it. Although the assessment process is ongoing, after you have collected some initial information about the current situation and dynamics, you will be ready to prepare an initial assessment write-up. The level of detail and the things on which you focus in your write-up will depend on the type of program, organizational or funder requirements, and other unique characteristics of your relationship with the family. Before you begin writing your assessment summary, think about how it will be used and who will read it. A good rule of thumb to follow is to write clearly, using your observations to support your discussion, and to write as if you are not available and someone else is picking up the case. I often suggest to new home visitors that they also

SIDEBAR 4.8

Sample Family Assessment Summary

I. Identifying information and initial presentation
   A. In this section, include identifying information such as ages of family members, sex, race, marital status, and a brief statement of the presenting problem.
II. Current situation
   A. Risks—Summarize the information on the Risk Factor Checklist.
   B. Current functioning—Describe the current living situation, and summarize items on the Checklist to Assess Current Functioning. Make sure you look at how the family is functioning and what their current stressors are.
   C. Social and environmental factors—Include a narrative summary of the ecomap and culturagram.
III. Developmental considerations and past history
   A. Describe relevant developmental and life history events. Include a discussion of how development and history are congruent or incongruent with cultural expectations.
IV. Available assessment data
   A. If you have psychological test results, diagnostic reports, responses to standardized instruments, information from the referral source, or any other additional information about the situation, summarize it here.
V. Summary
   A. Summarize your findings. Include a brief narrative regarding the readiness to change.

Remember, you want to provide enough detail so that if the family is assigned to someone else, the new staff member will have a good picture of what is going on. At the same time, avoid repeating yourself, be concise, and try to ground your assessment in observations rather than judgments or impressions.

SIDEBAR 4.9

Rodriguez Family Assessment

The Assessment

Over several weeks, Linda visited the Rodriguez family at their apartment. The following summaries of the family's risk and functioning, along with an ecomap are used to provide information for the assessment summary.

Risk Factor Checklist

Family: Rodriguez: Enrique, Silvia, Omar
Home Visitor: Linda Wilson

Score   Risk Factor

Score	Risk Factor	5	4	3	2	1
_1_	1. **Suicide**	high risk	considerable risk	moderate risk	slight risk	no risk/low risk
_1_	2. **Violent behavior**	high risk	considerable risk	moderate risk	slight risk	no risk/low risk
_3.5_	3. **Depression**	high risk	considerable risk	moderate risk	slight risk	no risk/low risk
_1_	4. **Psychosis**	high risk	considerable risk	moderate risk	slight risk	no risk/low risk
_3.5_	5. **Anxiety**	high risk	considerable risk	moderate risk	slight risk	no risk/low risk
_3_	6. **Alcohol abuse**	high risk	considerable risk	moderate risk	slight risk	no risk/low risk
_2_	7. **Drug abuse**	high risk	considerable risk	moderate risk	slight risk	no risk/low risk
_2_	8. **Domestic violence**	high risk	considerable risk	moderate risk	slight risk	no risk/low risk
_2_	9. **Child abuse**	high risk	considerable risk	moderate risk	slight risk	no risk/low risk
_NA_	10. **Elder abuse**	high risk	considerable risk	moderate risk	slight risk	no risk/low risk
_2_	11. **Overall risk**	high risk	considerable risk	moderate risk	slight risk	no risk/low risk

The overall level of current risk is slight.

SIDEBAR 4.9 *(continued)*

Current Functioning Checklist

Family: Rodriguez: Enrique, Silvia, Omar
Home Visitor: Linda Wilson

1. Start with how the individual or family is doing with respect to carrying out key activities of daily life.

Area of functioning	Level of functioning				
Relationships with family	1 Very low	**(2) Poor**	3 Adequate	4 Good	5 Excellent
Relationships in the community	1 Very low	**(2) Poor**	3 Adequate	4 Good	5 Excellent
School/work	1 Very low	**(2) Poor**	3 Adequate	4 Good	5 Excellent
Adequacy of role functioning	1 Very low	2 Poor	**(3) Adequate**	4 Good	5 Excellent
Coping and adaptive skills	1 Very low	**(2) Poor**	3 Adequate	4 Good	5 Excellent
Health	1 Very low	2 Poor	**(3) Adequate**	4 Good	5 Excellent
Self-care	1 Very low	2 Poor	**(3) Adequate**	4 Good	5 Excellent
Parenting	1 Very low	**(2) Poor**	3 Adequate	4 Good	5 Excellent

2. Now look at the severity of current stressors in the family's life.

Area of functioning	Level of problems				
Relationships with family	1 Significant	2 Noticeable	**(3) Moderate**	4 Mild	5 None
Relationships in the community	1 Significant	**(2) Noticeable**	3 Moderate	4 Mild	5 None
School/work	1 Significant	**(2) Noticeable**	3 Moderate	4 Mild	5 None
Adequacy of role functioning	1 Significant	2 Noticeable	**(3) Moderate**	4 Mild	5 None
Coping and adaptive skills	1 Significant	2 Noticeable	**(3) Moderate**	4 Mild	5 None
Health	1 Significant	2 Noticeable	**(3) Moderate**	4 Mild	5 None
Self-care	1 Significant	2 Noticeable	**(3) Moderate**	4 Mild	5 None
Parenting	1 Significant	**(2) Noticeable**	3 Moderate	4 Mild	5 None
Other NA	1 Significant	2 Noticeable	3 Moderate	4 Mild	5 None

Summary: Generally, the family is functioning at a poor to adequate level. Current stressors are noticeable, but somewhat moderate. The family is not in active crisis, but the overall level of functioning is low enough that an unexpected stressor might be more than they can easily manage.

SIDEBAR 4.9 *(continued)*

The Ecomap
Rodreguez Family

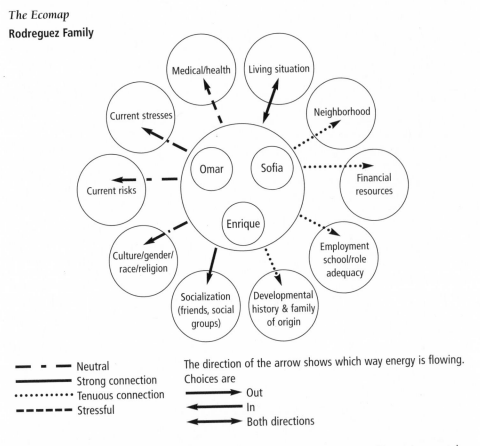

— - — Neutral
———— Strong connection
•••••••••• Tenuous connection
— — — — — Stressful

The direction of the arrow shows which way energy is flowing. Choices are
——→ Out
←—— In
←——→ Both directions

Summary: The ecomap indicates that the family has weak connections to most of its environmental, social, and personal support systems. While very few stressful relationships emerge, the family's energy generally is going out, with very little support or strong positive energy flowing in.

SIDEBAR 4.9 (*continued*)

Family Assessment Summary

Family: Rodriguez: Enrique, Silvia, Omar
Home Visitor: Linda Wilson

I. Identifying Information and Initial Presentation

A. Family members:
   1. Enrique, age twenty-nine, Latino male. Works as a laborer for several landscaping companies. Born in Mexico, citizenship status unknown.
   2. Sofia, age twenty-four, Latina female, housekeeper, currently working episodically. U.S. citizen.
   3. Omar, age eight months, male
B. Marital status is unknown at this time.
C. Presenting Problem: Baby exhibits chronic contagious skin infections, parents appear isolated, and there is some evidence of developmental and attachment concerns with the baby.

II. Current Situation

A. Risks: While the overall level of risk is slight, there is some elevated risk of depression, anxiety, and alcohol use.
B. Current Functioning: The family is functioning marginally. While they are not in active crisis, their resources are scarce, and their muted functioning may reduce resiliency in the event of a stressor.
C. Social and Environmental Factors: This is a fairly isolated young couple with few family or social resources. The ecomap indicates that the family is weakly connected to social and personal supports in the community. The family's housing is fairly stable, although they do not have adequate health care. Income is variable, and the family is struggling to keep up with their bills. The couple does not seem to be well connected to employment or educational opportunities and seems not to use cultural or community supports. Neither Enrique nor Sofia report any connection to religion, and report that they have very few friends.

III. Developmental Considerations and Past History

Enrique grew up in a Mexican family, spending time on both sides of the border. He indicates that family members were often concerned about deportation. His current immigration status is unknown, although he did attend several years of school in the U.S. He is not confident with his English, and prefers speaking Spanish. Enrique reports that he was the fourth of seven children, and that he often felt invisible in his family. His labor was necessary to help the family, but he does not report strong relationships among family members. His parents currently live across the border. He visits sporadically, but does not like to cross the border because he worries about having problems of some sort. He is vague about his concern, but does evidence general anxiety about getting into trouble with the authorities. Enrique reports that his childhood was uneventful, except for the death of his next younger sister. Enrique was five or six and does not know how she died, only that his mother went to bed for almost a year after his sister died. Enrique reports a dutiful, cordial relationship with his parents. He does not remember being hit or abused, although he does remember his father getting drunk sometimes and yelling a lot. Enrique left school in the eighth grade. He was in a U.S. school at the time, and failing. A friend's father helped Enrique find a job with a landscape company, and Enrique quit school to begin working. He lived at home and gave all of his money to his family. He met Sofia at a bar in a Mexican border city. They soon moved in together, on the U.S. side. Enrique still tries to send small amounts of money to his family, but it has become difficult since Sofia stopped working and he has to support his own family. Enrique indicates that he feels he is meeting his obligations as a husband, a father, and a son, but he does not understand why the nurse at the pediatrician's office always seems to disapprove of him and expect more from him.

Sofia is the oldest of three girls. Her father was unemployed and drank heavily. When she was fourteen he was arrested for smuggling narcotics across the border, and sentenced to prison. Sofia's mother cleaned houses and asked Sofia to start helping her out. Sofia's younger sister became pregnant when she was thirteen years old and now has three children, all of whom have been removed by child welfare services. Sofia's older sister is a methamphetamine addict, and was thrown out of the house by Sofia's mother when Sofia was fifteen. From the time that Sofia was fifteen until she met Enrique three years ago (about six years), Sofia lived with her mother. Sofia's mother depends heavily upon her emotionally, and until recently, financially. They have been in conflict since Omar's birth because Sofia's mother thinks that Sofia should be helping her out more. She cannot take care of Omar so Sofia can work, because the mother too must work and cannot afford the lost income. Sofia reports that her mother is somewhat childish and dependent, and that even when Sofia was a little girl she felt like she had to take care of her. Sofia describes her mother as someone who angers easily and holds a grudge. Sofia feels that she must find a way to help her mother financially. The mother's emotional support is limited because she seems to be preoccupied with her own problems. Sofia has lost all contact with her father.

IV. Available Assessment Data

A. The Parenting for Healthy Children Program utilizes several standardized screening instruments:
1. CES-D (Centers for Disease Control, Depression Scale): both Sofia and Enrique received scores indicating depression. Enrique's score indicates mild depression, while Sofia's score indicates more severe depression.[1]
2. MSS (Maternal Social Support Index) Score: the scores on the MSS were low, indicating very little support for the family.[2]
3. AAPI (Adult-Adolescent Parenting Inventory)[3] Both Sofia and Enrique scored low

on all dimensions of the AAPI. Especially noteworthy was Enrique's low scores on the dimensions associated with realistic expectations of children and belief in corporal punishment. Sofia scored quite low on the scale measuring the parent's ability to relate to the child empathetically.

The standardized screening instruments highlight the family's weak social supports, depression, and lack of knowledge about child development. The low empathy score, paired with the depression score for Sofia are notable.

V. Summary

This is a young family in need of a supportive social and community environment. Both parents seem to have had distant relationships with their own family members and are not knowledgeable about the needs of children. Both parents left school without obtaining a degree. Enrique is employed but receives no benefits, and Sofia works sporadically. They are struggling financially and are having trouble covering their own expenses and finding resources to send to their families. Sofia shows signs of depression, and the family, while not in crisis, seems unable to move ahead. Intimacy and attachment challenges affect the couple and their relationship with their baby, Omar. The baby is showing signs of troubled attachment and slow development.

1. Radloff, L. S. (1977). The CES-D scale: A self-report depression scale for research in the general population. Applied Psychological Measurement, 1, 385–401.

2. Pascoe, J. M., Ialongo, N. S., Horn, W. F., Reinhart, M. A., and Perrradatto, D. (1988). The reliability and validity of the Maternal Social Support Index. *Family Medicine* 271–76.

3. Bavolek, S. J., and Keene, R. G. (1999). *Handbook for the AAPI-2: Adult-Adolescent Parenting Inventory.* Park City, Utah: Family Development Resources.

write as if the families are looking over their shoulders; any impressions or opinions need to be clearly identified as such, and you should provide observational data to support what you have written. The assessment write-up should be clear, concise, and complete.

Depending upon your program, how it is funded, its mission, and the community and organizational context within which you are operating, there may be other dimensions beyond those described in this chapter that you will be asked to assess. The dimensions listed above will provide you with a good idea of the family, its strengths, and some of the challenges that you will face as you and family members try to move toward accomplishing their goals for change. Strengths-based assessments focus on the family's understanding of the problem, what brought it about, and what can be done about it. Ideally you and the family will come to a shared understanding of what is going on, how things got this way, and what needs to happen next.

SUMMARY

In this chapter we have explored some of the key considerations in completing a multidimensional assessment. The home visitor will need to attend to many factors regarding the ways in which the family and the context within which it is functioning interact with each other. Tools for capturing some of this data, such as a culturagram, ecomap, and risk assessment instrument are presented. Sometimes the family who is beginning its engagement with a program is in active crisis, and the home visitor will need to intervene in order to assure safety and help the family to be in a position receptive to change and growth. The home visitor is reminded to be highly sensitive to the processes and stages of change and to recognize how difficult it is for individuals and families to experience changes. We continue with the Rodriguez family, and in this chapter, some of the details of the family's initial assessment process are presented.

FIVE

Individualized Family Service Plan

The assessment summary provides the home visitor and the family with an outline of key issues and concerns. The next step involves identifying shared goals and developing a strategy to achieve those goals. The plan you develop with the family should address the family's unique concerns, strengths, and barriers. It serves as a guide to you and the family, and serves to keep the intervention focused.

WHAT IS AN INDIVIDUALIZED FAMILY SERVICE PLAN?

It is important to remember that even though many of the families you work with will articulate similar concerns and needs, they all got there following a unique, highly individualized path. For this reason you will need to focus on how to help *this family* with its unique experience of vulnerabilities, strengths, and solutions. Sometimes your program has a set menu of program services and options, and it is tempting to simply choose from the menu and get to work. This is especially true if the program is funded to carry out a particular model of home-visiting case management. These program options will be extremely helpful to you and the family as you develop a plan, but in and of themselves, they do not constitute a plan. It is important to individualize the service components to meet the family's goals and needs. If you have diligently worked

Figure 5.1 Individualized service plan

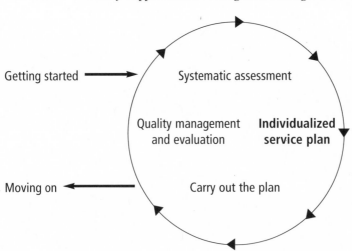

Family-Support Home-Visiting Case-Management Process

on developing an engagement with the family and have done a thorough assessment, you will have plenty of information to help you and the family to identify individualize strategies. The more the family feels that this is "their" plan, the more likely they are to carry out their part of it and to remain in the program. If family members feel that the plan is not theirs, it is likely they will not be highly committed to it. It is also likely that the family, especially if they are receiving services on a voluntary basis, will prematurely end the relationship if they do not feel that the services specifically address their concerns.

The individualized family service plan summarizes the activities you and the family plan to accomplish. It provides you and the family with a vision and a direction. Like assessments, plans represent an ongoing process that involves:

1. Rechecking the assessment information and adjusting goals if necessary.
2. Monitoring family responses to the strategy as it is carried out, and making adjustments to the plan as needed.
3. Identifying resources and barriers, both anticipated and unanticipated. There may be adjustments to the original plan based on new information.
4. Monitoring and utilizing the feedback obtained.

ESTABLISHING GOALS AND OBJECTIVES

The heart of the individualized family service plan centers on the goals and objectives. The goals are the outcomes that you and the family anticipate, and the objectives are the specific strategies that will be used to accomplish these goals. The goals flow out

---

SIDEBAR 5.1

The Planning Stage

Example of Goals, Objectives, and Activities

Goal: To Reduce Conflict in the Family (both frequency and intensity)

Objectives:

I. Identify "triggers."
   A. Activities:
      1. Family members will keep a journal of times that they lose their tempers.
      2. Family members will identify patterns.
II. Initiate alternative behaviors in "trigger" situations.
   A. Activities:
      1. Family members will agree upon signals to let others know that they are feeling stressed.
      2. Family members will agree upon a time-out arrangement (leaving the room, watching television, taking a walk) that each member can carry out before responding.
      3. After a time-out family members agree to carry on routine activities and record the conflict situation.
      4. Family members will review the circumstances of the conflict with a helping professional.
III. Reduce number of instances of yelling.
   A. Activities:
      1. Family members will try to use time-out behaviors before yelling.
      2. Family members will stop and count to ten before responding in conflict situations.
IV. Yelling episodes are shorter.
   A. Activities:
      1. Family members will jointly agree that if yelling breaks out the discussion will end for now.
      2. Family members will note the situation that led to yelling in their journal and discuss with a helping professional.

Note: These activities are tentative strategies agreed upon with the family. The home visitor will have

(Continued page 80)

Sample Individualized Family Service Plan Format[1]

Family:

Date of initial plan: Is this a revised/updated plan?   Date of revision:

Summary of goals to be accomplished:

1.

2.

3.

When will this plan be reviewed?

Goal to be accomplished	Strategies to accomplish	Specific activities and who will do them	Comments/evaluation of progress
1.	A. B. C.	1) 2) 3) 4) 5)	Describe what has been accomplished, any barriers or adjustments to time-lines or specific activities, any evalua-tion of progress
2.	A. B. C.	1) 2) 3) 4) 5)	
3.	A. B. C.	1) 2) 3) 4) 5)	

SIDEBAR 5.2 (*continued*)

Family members who will be part of the plan:

_____

I understand the plan and have been part of creating it. I will work with the home visitor to accomplish the goals and to review progress understand the plan and agree to it.

The home visitor has discussed confidentiality with me and I understand that this plan will be a confidential document.

Signature(s) of family member(s)   1. _____

2. _____

3. _____

4. _____

Home Visitor signature   _____

Plan will be reviewed (date)   _____

NOTES:

1. It is recommended that a copy of this form be given to the family so that they can refer to it regularly.

worked with the family to get a sense of realistic approaches to stopping the unwanted negative family interactions. The specific activities are best identified by family members. Therefore, the very same concerns in another family might be managed with a different set of objectives and activities. What is important here is that family members engage in identifying and addressing the things they are concerned about. These small incremental steps allow the family to partialize the problem and gain control over it in pieces. The home visitor supports the family's efforts, celebrates successes, and explores situations in which the strategy is not working. This exploration helps the family and home visitor to fine tune the strategy and keep the issue in the forefront. It also helps the family to see that the home visitor has confidence that the problem is resolvable, and that she/he has confidence in the family's capacity to come up with a solution. It should be clear that the goals, rather than being set immutably, are intended to undergo a constant process of refinement. The home visitor's ability to stay with the process, and maintain a positive attitude will help the family to gain confidence in their own ability to solve this and other problems.

of the assessment process. It is important to find out what issues are most important to the family and to help them prioritize and order goals. The goals should be: 1) clear, 2) specific, and 3) feasible. Vague, general goals will lose their meaning and may result in a loss of focus in your work with the family. Goals represent the positive expression of what family members would like to happen. The more goals are tied to specific, observable outcomes, the more likely they are to make sense to the family. Objectives describe the measurable strategies that will be used to accomplish goals. Objectives can be further broken down into specific activities.

WHERE DO THE GOALS AND OBJECTIVES COME FROM?

The goals that you and the family agree upon should be jointly established and take the following into consideration:

1. What the family says they would like to accomplish
2. What referral sources or outside mandating agencies want to see accomplished
3. Any standardized data, psychological tests, diagnostic information, or other assessment data
4. What you and your team think is needed to respond to the needs identified in the assessment

The primary consideration in establishing goals and objectives with a family has to do with what the family wants to accomplish. Teasing out the family's vision for itself and articulating specific goals is an important part of the planning process. Frequently, referring sources will recommend a course of action at the point of referral. This represents the referral source's assessment of the situation and what is needed. While this is important information, it should not dictate your action plan. This referral information is one piece of information that may help you and the family to identify working goals.

While data from test scores, standardized instruments, diagnostic workups, and other sources is helpful, it needs to be considered in the context of what the family is willing to do and their vision for themselves. Likewise, you and members of your team will form opinions about what might be helpful based on your interpretation of the assessment data. These ideas should be treated as tentative action steps that can be evaluated jointly with the family. It is important to treat the family as a partner in the process of establishing goals and a service plan. Rather than completing the assessment and deciding independently of the family that they need a particular set of interventions and services, it is preferable to share the assessment data with the family and work with them to understand the assessment and some possible goals and objectives that are responsive to the needs identified in the assessment. By engaging the family members as partners in the planning effort, you are more likely to encourage cooperation and follow through with the plan that is developed.

PREPARING A WORKING PLAN

Once you and the family have agreed upon the goals and objectives and the activities that you plan to use to accomplish them, it is important to prioritize the goals and to develop a timeline. Some goals will be very short-term and time limited, while others will be long-term and may involve a series of steps. It is sometimes helpful to think of these as "baby steps," since it may take the accomplishment of many small short-term goals to accomplish a large, long-term goal. The process of baby stepping is vital with overburdened families because many of them have developed a sense of helplessness and hopelessness. The idea of baby steps reflects the idea of self-efficacy. Efficacy theory indicates that the experience of success leads to the expectation of future success (Bandura 1994). In simple terms failure feeds on failure, and success builds further success. With this in mind it is urgent that the family service plan is a "live document," something that both you and the family refer to often, and adjust often. Small, doable steps are built in so that the family experiences success. One way to use the plan to build efficacy is to put it in a prominent place (the refrigerator is often a good place) and to remind family members frequently of what they have already accomplished. Remember, families who have come to expect failure will take time to recognize that they actually *CAN* do things that solve problems. For some individuals and families the experience of efficacy is so new that they need help recognizing that it is happening, and that they are, in fact, able to accomplish their goals.

In developing goals and objectives, it is useful to remember that the plan is always in process. That means that the initial goals are only a beginning and that as the relationship deepens and the family achieves some successes, new goals can be established. Over time the family's goals will evolve. Often the initial goals are fairly concrete and address immediate concerns. Over time the family may identify new goals, and the goals may become more complex and comprehensive. For instance, early in the home-visiting process, it may be necessary to help the family avoid eviction due to financial problems. Later, as housing and financial situations become more manageable, family members may find that they are interested in developing more supportive, nurturing relationships within the family. One way to think about this is to consider Maslow's idea of a hierarchy of needs. Maslow recognized that in order for people to be psychologically open to what he called self-actualization, it is necessary that their basic needs be met first. For this reason the home visitor will want to assure that survival and safety needs are adequately addressed. Maslow suggested the following hierarchy of needs (1954):

1. Basic survival and physical needs
2. Safety and security
3. Social belonging
4. Self-esteem
5. Self-actualization

Because overburdened families are often vulnerable to changes in living situations, income, and other basic needs, the home visitor will need to remain aware of these needs during the assessment, and for the duration of the helping relationship with the family. Family situations can be precarious, and the plan should take into account the family's need to develop as much stability as possible.

The family service plan will need to be tailored to the specific circumstances of each family and should incorporate goals that you and the family have identified and agreed to work toward. The following template is a guide to help you prepare an individualized family service plan. It is important to try to be as detailed and specific as possible regarding what will be done and who will do it. The finished plan serves as an agreement between you and the family and is something that will guide your work, and later, your evaluation of your effectiveness. The family uses the plan to evaluate their accomplishment of important goals.

SPECIALIZED PLANS

At times you will want to develop specialized plans to address specific issues such as child safety, domestic violence safety planning, maintenance planning, and crisis prevention planning. These tend to be risk related, or to address circumstances in which a family member is working to maintain new behaviors and avoid relapses. These specialized plans need to be specific and related directly to the problem of concern. Sidebar 5.3 gives an example of a maintenance plan. The specialized plan can be used to highlight a concern and help family members to prioritize risk reduction goals. It should be considered ancillary to the overall family service plan.

Sidebar 5.4 provides an illustration of an individualized family service plan for the Rodriguez family. Note that the initial summary includes a discussion of what the family and the home visitor have agreed to, and includes some of the considerations raised by the home visitor's supervisor and team. With a basic agreement about what is to be done, the home visitor and the family then moved to a discussion of the specific action steps that would be needed to accomplish the goals.

SUMMARY

In this chapter we have examined the way a family service plan is developed. The plan includes goals identified by the family and home visitor, and utilizes data from referral

---
■

SIDEBAR 5.3

Sample Specialized Plan—Maintenance Plan[2]

Family: Brown, Freda (mother) and George (father); Sharon (daughter), Michael (son)
Date: March 5, 2005

What is the concern?

Freda becomes overwhelmed, loses her temper, and says hurtful things to other family members, and sometimes hits Sharon. Freda has been taking medications and is in counseling. Her outbursts have become infrequent, but the family worries about preventing and managing future incidents.

What will each family member do if an incident is starting or about to happen?

Freda: Recognize triggers
           Take a time out
           Call a designated friend
           Contact the mental health counselor
           Take medications regularly
           Will remind herself that her family loves her and is not the enemy
George: Will not take Freda's outbursts personally and will take a time out if necessary
           Help Freda remember to take her medications
           Offer to handle the kids if Freda is losing control
           Will protect the children by leaving the house if necessary
Sharon: Will call her father or the neighbor if things escalate with Mom
           Will not yell back but will go to her room and take a time out
           If necessary, will leave the house and go to the neighbor's
           Will call 911 if she cannot contact father or neighbor
Michael: Will call her father or the neighbor if Mom is yelling
           Will not whine and cry for attention when mom is yelling at Sharon
           If necessary, will leave the house and go to the neighbor's
           Will call 911 if he cannot contact father or neighbor

If the children are alone and Freda becomes abusive they will call:

1. Dad (619) 240–7859
2. Mrs. Morgan (619) 245–0799
3. 911

George will notify his employer that if his children call, it is an emergency and he may need to take care of business at home.

If Freda begins an incident and is able to stop herself, all family members will acknowledge her success.

Family members will hold a family meeting once a week to discuss how the week went.

I understand the plan and have been part of creating it. I will work with the home visitor to accomplish the goals, to review progress, understand the plan, and agree to it. The home visitor has discussed confidentiality with me and I understand that this plan will be a confidential document.

Family Signatures/Date
_____

_____
Home Visitor Signature/Date

2. This plan is specific to this family, and has been worked out with family members to address a concern of theirs. This is not the complete family service plan, but instead, highlights a specific area upon which the family needs and wants to focus. A copy should be made for the family to keep handy.

sources, professional knowledge, and objective assessments, as well as from the family's own experiences. The plan needs to take into account the importance of first meeting basic needs, and must be constructed in such a way that it is doable. The family and the home visitor will need to focus on specific, small increments that are achievable.

SIDEBAR 5.4

Rodriguez Family Individualized Family Service Plan

Family: Rodriguez: Enrique, Silvia, Omar

Home Visitor: Linda Wilson

Date: January 23, 2005

The home visitor considered the following information in working with the family to develop a plan:

1. *What Sofia and Enrique say they want*

Enrique indicated that he wanted to learn more English and get a GED so he could become a supervisor at a landscaping company and perhaps receive health care benefits. Sofia indicated that she wants to go back to work, but is afraid to leave Omar in anyone's care. Both Enrique and Sofia wanted help meeting their obligations to their families.

2. *What the home visitor and family-support case-management team thinks needs to happen*

The team and the home visitor would like to see both parents receive degrees and perhaps some job training so that they can find more stable employment. A number of team members felt that the couple needed to free itself of the sense of financial obligation to their families, but others felt that for cultural reasons it would be inappropriate for Sofia and Enrique to ignore this responsibility. All team members felt that Sofia's depression and issues of intimacy and attachment should be addressed. The team also felt that Omar's development was at risk and that a specialized child development intervention might be needed. The team also felt that the couple needed to become more connected to resources in the community, such as a church. The team also felt that the couple might want to look for activities at the local recreation center where they might meet other people.

3. *What the assessment data show*

The assessment data show some concern about depression, connection to supportive community resources, and a need to develop more intimacy between Enrique and Sofia. The data show a need for help with understanding how to bond with and parent baby Omar.

The goals

After reviewing the assessment with Enrique and Sofia, and sharing some of the home visitor and team's ideas, Linda asked Enrique and Sofia with which goals they would like to start. Initially the plan was focused on helping Enrique to learn English and obtain his GED. Later the couple became very interested in learning more about parenting. Still later they became interested in working on their own relationship and their relationships with family members. Eventually Sofia felt the need to address her depression and became interested in obtaining her GED. Toward the end of the three-year period both Enrique and Sofia became interested in working on building friendships in the community. The following plan was the first one established between the home visitor and the Rodriguez family.

SIDEBAR 5.4 (*continued*)

Individualized Family Service Plan

Family: Rodriguez

Date of initial plan: Jan. 2   **Is this a revised/updated plan?** New plan   **Date of revision:**

Summary of goals to be accomplished:

1. Enrique will enroll in ESL classes.
2. Enrique will enroll in a GED program.
3. Plan will be reviewed and decision to continue will be made.

Goal to be accomplished	Strategies to accomplish	Specific activities and who will do them	Comments/evaluation of progress
1. Enrique will enroll in ESL classes.	A. Identify nearby ESL classes. B. Identify scheduling needs. C. Identify transportation and financing needs. D. Choose an ESL program and enroll. E. Program will be completed.	1. Linda will identify ESL resources and discuss with Enrique. 2. Enrique, Sofia, and Linda will review times, locations, fees, and other logistics. 3. The family will weight the options and pick a program that best fits schedule, location, and other logistic needs. 4. Linda will go with Enrique to enroll in the program. 5. Enrique will attend classes and complete the program.	Enrique and Sofia needed assistance with working out the logistics. We needed to review the time he gets off work, how long it takes to get to each location, and ease of transportation home. Additionally Enrique needed to pack extra food to bring with him for dinner. Sofia developed a plan to structure her evening, since it became clear that she was going to be alone on school nights after having been alone all day. She decided to use her time knitting and crocheting items for the family. Enrique found that he was very tired and needed encouragement to continue. Linda helped Sofia obtain transportation for herself and Omar so that she could attend the ceremony when Enrique obtained his certificate. (March 2—)

Goal to be accomplished	Strategies to accomplish	Specific activities and who will do them	Comments/evaluation of progress
2. Enrique will enroll in a GED program.	A. Identify nearby GED classes. B. Identify scheduling needs. C. Identify transportation and financing needs. D. Choose a GED program and enroll. E. Program will be completed.	1. Linda will identify GED resources and discuss with Enrique. 2. Enrique, Sofia and Linda will review times, locations, fees, and other logistics. 3. The family will weight the options and pick a program that best fits schedule, location and other logistic needs. 4. Linda will go with Enrique to enroll in the program. 5. Enrique will attend classes and receive his GED.	By now (June 2—), Enrique has the schedule, transportation, and other logistics well under control. He struggles with some of the subjects, but continues to attend the program. Sofia has begun sewing placemats that she sells to a neighbor. The neighbor sells the placements in a tourist area and pays Sofia a small amount. The family plans a small party when Enrique receives his GED. Family members are invited, and some come. The neighbor prepares food and attends the celebration.
3. Plan will be reviewed, and a decision to continue or not will be made.	After Enrique completes the ESL program and the GED, the family will meet with Linda to determine if they feel they have completed their goals or would like to continue working together.	As the time nears for Enrique to obtain his GED, Linda begins exploring with the family their intentions. Several sessions are spent reviewing progress so far.	It appears that new goals are emerging. The family wants to work on finding Enrique a better job, perhaps as a supervisor in a landscape company. Sofia wants to learn how to deal with Omar's temper (he is now approaching 2 years), and shows some interest in rejoining the parenting classes.

SIDEBAR 5.4 (*continued*)

Family members who will be part of the plan: Enrique, Sofia

I understand the plan and have been part of creating it. I will work with the home visitor to accomplish the goals and to review progress understand the plan and agree to it. The home visitor has discussed confidentiality with me and I understand that this plan will be a confidential document.

Signature(s) of family member(s)	Enrique Rodriguez
	Sofia Rodriguez
Home Visitor signature	Linda Wilson
Plan will be reviewed (date)	March, June, Sept 2—

NOTES:

It appears that as the original goals are met the family has identified additional goals and is ready to continue services, including working on parenting skills.

SIX

Carrying Out the Plan

After developing a tentative service plan with the family and obtaining their agreement to carry it out, the home visitor is faced with following through with and sustaining the specific actions that will be needed to carry out the plan. It is important to keep in mind that the family will need your help in remaining focused on the goals of the plan.

Figure 6.1 Carrying out the plan

Family-Support Home-Visiting Case-Management Process

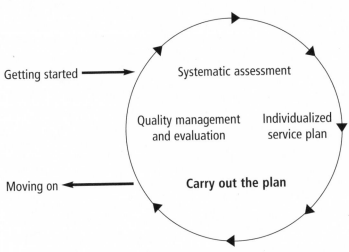

Many overburdened families will need help recognizing themselves as being in control of the things that happen in their lives. What this means is that even though they have formed a plan with you, it is likely that the family will wait for something to happen or for you to DO something. An important part of empowering families is helping them to recognize that they in fact have the ability and the power to carry out the activities that will help them function better and solve the problems that brought them to your agency. Often members of vulnerable families have tried things in the past and have become discouraged. Over time they have become convinced that there is nothing they can do and they are at the mercy of agencies, courts, schools, and other social institutions they do not always understand completely. This is an example of learned helplessness (Seligman 1975). An important part of the home visitor's job is to interrupt this cycle and begin to reverse it by offering the family opportunities to build a sense of efficacy. Health, interpersonal, and social problems are reduced as family members become better able to problem solve, exercise good judgment, and consistently move toward their goals. These skills are developed through experiences and feedback from others. The home visitor is working with family members to improve their abilities to sort out and prioritize problems, identify and evaluate potential action strategies, carry out those strategies, and build new patterns of behavior through practice and reflection.

Efficacy comes from building upon small successes. Each time family members are able to set a goal, establish a strategy, and carry out that strategy, their sense of being able to control their lives will be increased. Part of the home visitor's challenge is helping the family to stay focused on accomplishing the small steps and celebrating each accomplishment, no matter how small.

The human tendency is to look at the big goal and to discount the small steps along the way. For instance, high school graduation is a goal for many family members. However, this large goal needs to be broken down into smaller, more manageable pieces. For example, in order to graduate from high school, one needs to pass certain courses. Often the vulnerable, overburdened individual appears resistant or disinterested because he/she attends irregularly, is late, is not prepared, is tired, or in other ways is not able to perform consistently. The home visitor, using a strengths-based perspective might look at this and recognize that the individual needs assistance with the skills of developing a behavioral structure and maintaining it. If

SIDEBAR 6.1

Home Visitor Reflections

- Listen carefully to family members and find out about their feelings and needs. Exhibit respect, acceptance, and empathy.

- Do not be too gullible. Listen carefully and respectfully, but explore things you have doubts about.

- Be patient. Change is difficult and people move at their own pace. Progress can be very slow, and it is important not to push too hard for change.

- Be prepared for setbacks and disappointments. Do not judge or reject family members when things don't go as planned. They are used to rejection. Your ability to stay connected to the family even when there is a crisis or disappointment may be very new for them. These setbacks can actually strengthen your relationship with the family if you are able to stick with them through some of the difficult periods. It will help the family to experience continuity and security in the relationship, and this, in turn, will help them as they try to change.

- Do not do for the family what they can do for themselves. Help family members to think through their problems and find ways to stimulate them to discover their own solutions. As the family gains experience with successful problem resolution, they will gain confidence in their coping abilities.

- Do not let multiple or complex problems overwhelm you. Help the family members to sort out concerns and address each one individually. While working on one issue, resist the distraction of another problem.

- Be aware of the family's strengths and do not just pay attention to weaknesses and problems. They probably have heard enough about their deficits. Emphasize the positives—these are the building blocks of success.

- Try not to jump to conclusions. Stop, explore, and think about it before you come to a quick conclusion.

an individual has not had the opportunity to learn some very basic time management and planning skills, he/she may require skill building in these areas.

Figure 6.2 Building efficacy one step at a time

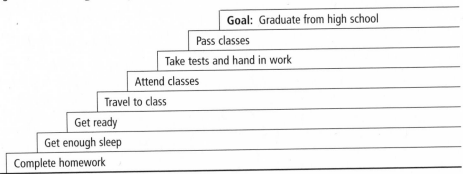

If we return to the example of setting high school graduation as a goal, it becomes clear that in order to pass courses, one needs to understand the material, pass tests, and accomplish the required work. In order to complete the required work, one needs to be rested, arrive at classes regularly, and engage with the course material. Thus the home visitor may need to work backward and identify all of the steps necessary to get to the final goal. It is not unusual that the home visitor and the family would need to spend time developing a plan for going to bed and waking up on time. Additionally a plan to structure the morning so that the individual, in coordination with other family members, can get dressed, eat breakfast, and travel to classes might require time and attention. It is easy to dismiss these small, mundane tasks, but without them, the steps along the way to goal accomplishment become impossible. It is important to remind yourself and the family that the sometimes-maddening attention to detail is an important part of getting there.

An important component of building new skills is the relationship between the home visitor and the family. The home visitor provides a consistent holding environment that serves as a secure place for the client to openly explore new ideas and behaviors. The nonjudgmental, safe relationship environment is also essential so that the family member can return for support and emotional rebuilding if things do not go well. Many overburdened families face maturational struggles. That is, the parents and other family members may not have had the opportunity to achieve important developmental tasks related to cognitive and emotional structuring. They may have struggled with less than optimal attachment experiences, and may not have successfully negotiated the social and emotional tasks associated with developing trust, autonomy, and initiative (Erickson 1963). Recent brain research has shown that there are critical periods in development that actually result in brain structures that are reflected in progressively more organized problem solving and interaction behavior. However, many vulnerable families require assistance with remediation and with reopening developmental activities.

At this juncture, it is important to remind ourselves that family-support home visiting is a generalized therapeutic intervention at the same time that it is not, strictly speaking, a therapy. The development of a relationship that permits the family members to reflect and revisit their own maturational gaps allows the family to identify and develop new skills. The development of these skills is therapeutic, in that it improves the family's internal relationships as well as its relationship with the community context within which it is situated. As a home visitor, you are expected to be therapeutic, yet you are not usually providing therapy in the traditional sense.

An additional consideration that will shape your work with a family has to do with recognizing and understanding their cultural practices and traditions. It is important that your home visits fit into a pattern that is comfortable for the family and for you. Make it a point to find out how the family feels about important things like being on time, physical proximity, and touching or speaking to children or other family members. Cultural ideas about offering food and accepting gifts can provide significant challenges to maintaining professional boundaries. Program directors and

> **SIDEBAR 6.2**
>
> ## What the Home Visitor Does
>
> - Establishes a consistent "holding environment"
> - Develops a trusting relationship with the family
> - Demonstrates cultural competency
> - Maintains contact and continuity, no matter what—stays engaged
> - Maintains confidentiality
> - Uses good communications and relationship skills
> - Builds family efficacy
>   - Helps the family break down or "partialize" problems
>   - Keeps the family focused on the small steps and reminds them that each step leads toward the big goal
> - Pays close attention to the goals in the family service plan and checks in regularly with the family to assess progress and assure that the goals are still relevant
> - Practices new skills with the family
> - Helps the family rehearse new skills
> - Always follows through with commitments and promises
> - Provides a bridge to services and resources
> - Communicates hope to the family

supervisors may find the following examples helpful as training tools. Home visitors may want to read them and think about how they might respond.

The Aldrondo Family

You have been working with the Aldrondo family for nine months providing home-visiting services. The family had a premature infant and several other children. You were able to help them prioritize the many crises they were experiencing, and they are now using community supports well and managing things in the family much better than before. The family is clearly feeling more in control of things, and is very grateful for your help. At a routine home visit the family offers you a present, a large photograph of the children in a beautiful, expensive frame. What would you do?

1. Accept the present.
2. Protest that you cannot accept such a present.
3. Ask if they have a smaller picture.
4. Tell them that your agency policy does not allow you to accept gifts.
5. Do something else (describe)

While there is not a single "correct" response, there are some difficult considerations associated with each option. The home visitor should review the situation with his or her supervisor and work with the supervisor to find a response that enhances the client's efficacy and creates a sense of mutuality.

The Black Bear Family

You are working with a Native American family, who lives in a very remote area. You have just started providing home-visiting services to a young mother who has given birth to twins, one of whom has died. The remaining twin is frequently ill and is likely to have some motor problems because of birth asphyxia. On one visit with the young mother, you notice an older man in the room. He is quiet and does not seem to notice your presence even though you greet him as you enter. Your client explains that this is her grandfather. What would you do?

1. Accept what she says and do not mention it further.
2. Ask her how he feels about your visits.
3. Ask if he understands what is being discussed and how this is for her.
4. Try to talk to the gentleman and engage him in the conversation.
5. Do something else. (describe)

While there is not a specific response that is "correct," the home visitor should try to understand the ways in which the identified client perceives the presence of the older man. Taking the client's lead will allow the home visitor to incorporate the older gentleman in a way that is culturally appropriate, should the client and her grandfather indicate that this is their intention in having him present.

The Shirii Family

You have been assigned to the Shirii family. The family is originally from Iran. The parents have been in the United States for over twenty-five years and have come to your program asking for help with Josh, their adolescent son. Mr. and Mrs. Shirii are quiet and unassuming people and do not know how to handle their son's rebelliousness. He is not doing his schoolwork and has been arrested once for breaking into a local store after-hours. They have asked for help with discipline and in understanding child development. When you arrive, Mrs. Shirii is dressed formally and has set out a teapot and plates of fruits, nuts, and pastries. What would you do?

1. Sit down and begin the visit without mentioning the food.
2. Indicate that you notice the food, but have just had your lunch and are not hungry.
3. Tell her that your agency has a policy against accepting food from clients.
4. Accept the food and eat it during the visit, along with the Shirii's.
5. Do something else. (describe)

The family's culture dictates that food be offered to visitors, and it is expected that guests will partake in some way. If the program works with many clients from this culture, it is suggested that policies be prepared in advance for such circumstances. While there are many reasons to be hesitant about taking food from families, the home visitor might put a small amount on a plate and take a few bites in order to avoid insulting the family. Since this situation will recur with this family, it is possible to review the issues with your supervisor or team and develop a plan for managing the situation in future interactions.

It should be obvious by now that there is not necessarily a set "correct" response for each situation. A great deal depends upon the policies of the program. Ideally the program will develop policies about gifts and food that can serve as guidelines for staff. Developing cultural competence is a lifelong undertaking. Most programs offer training in cultural competence, but you will need to pay attention to your own development in this area as well. A culturally competent person is one who recognizes and understands a number of different cultural paradigms and possesses a good understanding of his/her own cultural values and assumptions. Families need to feel confident that you understand what is important to them and that you respect their traditions. At the same time, it is reassuring for them to know that you are comfortable with who you are. Home visitors need to adapt their interventions and engagement styles in response to clients' cultural expectations. Class, ethnicity, and personal history can play an important role in the way that family members experience and utilize cultural values. Even when you are of a similar ethnic group, or have a great deal of familiarity with a particular ethnic group, it is necessary to understand the particular ways in which family members understand their cultural values. The family is going to engage and interact in a way that is consistent with their cultural values and it is important for you to be able to understand them in a way that does not presuppose that difference is pathological.

SIDEBAR 6.3

Home Visitor Skills

- **Questions:** Use open-ended questions and try to explore the family member's meaning in detail.
- **Empathy:** Put yourself in the family member's place. How would you be feeling if the things the family member is experiencing were happening to you?
- **Wondering:** This is a good way to introduce an idea or suggestion in a way that allows the family member to consider it without feeling obligated to accept it. Be tentative. Avoid being too authoritative or certain about things. Being too definitive can create resistance. "I am wondering if you have thought of any ways to help Ricky feel comfortable when you take him to his new school?"
- **Specific feedback:** This can be an effective way to shape behavior. "I notice you have been responding very honestly to Sally when she asks about her dad."
- **Normalizing:** Try to show the family that their experience is similar to others. Be careful not to minimize or to deny the uniqueness of the family's experiences. This technique can be very encouraging, since it helps family members to feel less isolated and different. "Lots of children who have had these experiences worry so much about being good that they become very anxious. John is doing this now. We will be working together to help him with this."
- **Ask, do not tell.** Asking allows the family to maintain a sense of being in control and permits them to exercise self-determination. "This is a group to help parents who want to know more about their child's development. Would you be interested in attending?"
- **Openness:** The family's class, culture, religion, and unique history affect the ways they perceive and respond to events. The home visitor strives to understand the unique and particular experience of the family.

■───────────────

SIDEBAR 6.4

Structure of the Home Visit

I. Beginning
   A. Break the ice, establish (or reestablish) rapport.
   B. Start where the client is today, including assessing functioning and current risk.
   C. Review prior visit and set goals for today's visit.
II. Middle
   A. Review the service plan and explore how it is progressing. Discuss any changes, barriers, or new opportunities that have emerged.
   B. Use active listening, engagement, and communication skills.
   C. Carry out the activities that you and the family had agreed upon (depending upon what is going on this may be interrupted by new events or crises, but as much as possible try to do what you said you would.
III. End
   A. Review the visit and overall progress—summarize the visit.
   B. Remind the family of any upcoming appointments, and review any specialized plans you and the family may have developed.
   C. Agree upon any activities to take place in the interim.
   D. Encourage feedback/reflection about the visit.
   E. Remind the family of how they can contact you and reinforce the date, time, and planned activities for the next meeting.
   F. Say goodbye.

(Continued on facing page)

Sometimes the solutions that make sense to you will be too far removed from the family's cultural norms, and therefore, it is important to learn enough about the family's culture to help them identify solutions that are culturally appropriate.

STRUCTURING YOUR VISITS

It is important to organize each visit so that you and the family can be sure that everything will get done. It is a good idea to establish some rituals that the family can count on. For instance, you might start each visit with a similar phrase, such as: "So, how has the past week been?" By establishing a routine that the family can count on, you will be helping them to gain comfort with the relationship. From the safety of a relationship that is predictable and can be counted upon, the family can more easily consider and practice new problem solving approaches.

Every visit will have a beginning, middle, and end, and you will need to carry out any follow-up activities in the interim between visits.

Beginning

Remember, many overburdened families are not accustomed to consistent relationships they can count on. It is usually a good idea to use the first few minutes to reconnect with the family and do a quick assessment of what is going on right now for the family. You might even consider setting up a routine with the family in which you jointly review the week during the first part of your visit. You can use this review to determine if any crises are emerging, adjust your plan for the rest of today's visit, and get a picture of how the family is progressing. Although you might have come prepared with a plan for today's visit, it is important to determine where the family is. Your plan may need to be adapted based on issues that are pressing or events that have transpired since your last visit. After a quick review and assessment of the family's current needs and pressures, it is a good idea to end this initial phase of the visit with a review of what they have shared with you. With the family you can then establish an agenda and goals for today's visit. It is a good idea to try to tie today's agenda back to the service plan and to items that were discussed in previous visits.

Middle

During this part of the visit you and the family will work through the agreed upon agenda and work toward meeting the goals of the service plan. During this part of the visit you will explore the family's progress

> IV. Follow Through
>   A. Document the visit.
>   B. Review with your supervisor/team.
>   C. Self-reflection and identification of concerns, possible countertransference, and other areas in which you will need support.
>   D. Develop some tentative ideas about the scope of your work with the family.
>   E. Carry out any referrals or other activities that you agreed to.

in more depth and explore any barriers they might be encountering. With the family you will be able to analyze barriers, questions, and concerns they may have, and begin to identify ways to move forward. During the middle stage, you and the family will be following up on activities in the plan. You will also be exploring the family's responses to the things they are doing related to the service plan and problem solving with them to try to keep things moving forward.

End

It is important for the family to know they can count on you to structure the visits. Ending on time provides them with some clear structure and allows both you and the family to plan your time together. The home visitor signals that the end of the visit is approaching and begins a review with the family of what has happened today, what next steps have been identified, and what to expect in the next visit. As the visit is ending, you and the family should agree upon what each of you will do before the next visit. You may want to remind the family about how they can contact you, and remind them of any specialized plans that are in place. The ending ritual should reassure the family that they can count on your return and help them to hold both themselves and you accountable for agreed-upon activities. As you close the visit you extend the continuity of the relationship by reminding the family that there will be continued contact.

Follow Through

After the visit it is important to make notes about what you and the family have agreed to do in the interim. You will also want to record what happened in today's visit and review the visit with your supervisor or team. If you find you have questions about such things as boundaries, the relationship with the family, and frustrations with progress, or if you need resources or information, make a note of this so you can review these questions in supervision. Make sure you follow up on the things you told the family you would do and prepare a tentative plan for your next visit.

By trying to maintain a structure for every visit, it will be easier to maintain focus and continuity. Write a brief outline of your plan for each session before you meet with

───────────────────────────────■───────────────────────────────

SIDEBAR 6.5

Home Visit Plan Checklist ·

Date: _____   Family: _____

Home visitor: _____

Before the Visit

☐   Review key issues from last visit. (Briefly note)

☐   What follow-up is needed? (Briefly note)

☐   Have I done all of the things that I said I would at our last visit? (Briefly note)

☐   What goals from the service plan are we working on today? (Describe)

☐   Are there any smaller goals/successes that we need to review and celebrate this visit? (Describe)

☐   What activities will we carry out today? (Include items you specifically plan to review or discuss with the family)

☐   Who am I expecting to participate in today's visit? (List the participants)

☐   What do I need to bring? (List the items you need to bring to the visit, such as forms, food, diapers, brochures, learning aides, toys, and so on)

☐   What are some of the key issues of concern to the family? (List concerns such as domestic violence, substance abuse, mental health concerns, child development, health, and so on)

After the Visit

☐   Any questions or concerns? (Describe briefly)

☐   Did I agree to carry out any activities or follow up with anything? (Describe)

☐   What did we agree to do at the next visit?

Notes:

∎

SIDEBAR 6.6

Home Visit Plan Checklist

Date: Feb., 2— (3rd visit)   **Family:** Rodriguez

Home visitor: Linda Wilson

Before the Visit

☒ Review key issues from last visit. (Briefly note)
Enrique tried to enroll at the local adult school ESL classes, but they had already started and he was not permitted to enroll. He is discouraged and feels we are just wasting time now.

☒ What follow-up is needed? (Briefly note)
I agreed to see if classes are offered at another location. I found a class, but it involves travel (gas $). We may have to review the budget to accommodate the added cost. I also agreed to bring some coupons for diapers that we have.

☒ Have I done all of the things I said I would at our last visit? (Briefly note)
Yes

☒ What goals from the service plan are we working on today? (Describe)
We will continue to work on ESL classes. Today we will problem solve time and budget issues related to the class. I will also be working to help Sofia play with the baby by bringing some toys.

☒ Are there any smaller goals/successes we need to review and celebrate this visit? (Describe)
Need to remind family that the first step was going to the adult school. Refocus on goal of ESL and remind them there are alternatives.

☒ What activities will we carry out today? (Include items that you specifically plan to review or discuss with the family)
We'll review Enrique's disappointment and frustration and work on getting him enrolled at the alternative site.

☒ Who am I expecting to participate in today's visit? (List the participants)
Primarily Enrique and Sofia. The baby will also be present.

☒ What do I need to bring? (List the items you need to bring to the visit, such as forms, food, diapers, brochures, learning aides, toys, and so on)
I will be bringing coupons and some toys for the baby. I will also bring the registration materials for the ESL class and help Enrique fill them out.

☒ What are some of the key issues of concern to the family? (List concerns such as: domestic violence, substance abuse, mental health concerns, child development, health, and so on)
The family wants to work on improving their situation by having Enrique learn more English and obtain a GED. I am concerned about the baby and will be encouraging more interaction through modeling.

After the Visit

☒ Any questions or concerns? (Describe briefly)
Although the family did not mention child development issues when we did the plan, I am concerned that Enrique and Sofia do not know much about development and need to be

SIDEBAR 6.6 *(continued)*

taught to play with Omar and talk to him. I don't know how to introduce this, since the couple is not focused on the baby, but on their own development.

☒ Did I agree to carry out any activities or follow up with anything? (Describe)
   I agreed to accompany Enrique to the first ESL class—Tuesday.

What did we agree to do at the next visit?

We will review how the first class went, including how Sofia felt being left alone, and how expensive gas was.

Notes:

Need to talk to the team about getting the parents more involved with the baby and helping them to communicate and play with him. Need help.

---

the family. Make sure your plan incorporates their goals from the family service plan and regularly remind them of the progress they are making. Sometimes you might want to review the small steps that have been accomplished and reinforce the idea that things are moving in the right direction. Your ability to focus attention on the big picture at the same time that you work in a very detailed way on the small steps leading to the big picture will provide modeling and encouragement to the family.

SUMMARY

In this chapter we have reviewed the nuts and bolts of carrying out the home-visiting plan. The home visitor is encouraged to focus on small goals and to celebrate small gains with the family. Understanding the ways that the family's culture affects engagement and the relationship with the home visitor is important. The home visitor will need to structure his or her visits and maintain a structure to the contacts in order to continue progressing toward the accomplishment of the goals set with the family.

SEVEN

Moving On and Ending Services

The relationship with the family changes and develops over time. The family-support home visitor and the family may expand or change the initial goals, and new events may affect the service plan and working relationship. In any event there comes a time when the home visitor and the family decide separately, or together, that it is time to move on. This stage of the case-management process is sometimes called ending, discharge, or termination. From a strengths perspective, it is recommended that you think of this stage as a graduation or a moving on to new things.

Figure 7.1 Moving on

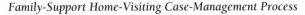

Family-Support Home-Visiting Case-Management Process

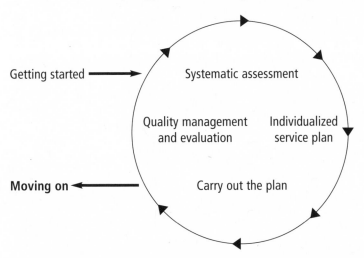

It is important for both the home visitor and the family to have a sense of closure as the family moves on. This is the end of a process and a transition to new things for the family. How the family experiences the process of transition can be very important to their future openness to seeking support and help with problem solving. "Closure . . . is a process in which practitioners and clients bring their work to a mutually understood (not necessarily satisfactory) end, review their work together (successes and failures), perhaps acknowledge feelings about the relationship, and acquire an enhanced willingness to invest in future relationships" (Walsh 2003, 5).

REASONS FOR MOVING ON

There are many reasons to initiate the transitional process leading to a family's moving on to new relationships and completing a process of closure with you. Here are some common reasons that families move on.

1. Mutual Agreement

The home visitor and the family mutually recognize and agree that the originally agreed upon goals have been achieved. In this case the family and the home visitor mutually agree that the family-support home-visiting intervention has gone as far as it can, and it is time for the family to make a transition to other resources or to try on their own to use the skills they have learned.

2. Time Limits

Many programs operate within a time frame that can range from a few weeks to several years. The home visitor must honor the parameters of the program funding or the intervention model that is supported by his/her organization. This time limit should be an important part of your work with the family from the beginning and can serve to help you and the family to stay focused and to prioritize activities. Shortly before the time limit is reached, you and the family will need to begin talking about the process of closure and planning for a transition.

3. Eligibility Changes

Similar to the limitations of funding and time limits, there may be eligibility criteria that are no longer met. These can be such things as moving to a new geographical area that is no longer covered by your program, reaching a certain age, entering school, or any other change in the family's status that affects whether they meet the eligibility criteria for your program. Families who have been court ordered or otherwise mandated to accept services may need to transition to another program at the end of the mandate, or they may choose to end services now that they are no longer required to participate.

4. Home Visitor Availability

Home visitors cannot stay in the same job forever for a number of reasons. Changes in the home visitor's availability may be caused by a variety of things:

- promotions or reassignment within the organization
- obtaining a new job with another organization
- moving because of a spouse or partner's job
- pregnancy
- health concerns

While this is not an exhaustive list of all of the reasons that a home visitor might no longer be available to a family, the point is that the home visitor is for some reason not able to maintain a connection to the family in order to complete the agreed upon goals.

5. Family Dissatisfaction or Lack of Interest

Families may find that the relationship is not what they expected, or they may find they are not as interested in working on the concerns that were identified in the assessment and service planning process. Families may not like some things about the home visitor or the program, and may decide to end the relationship. Family members may become frustrated or disappointed, and while there is always the hope that these issues can be worked through, sometimes they cannot and the family chooses to leave the relationship.

Whether the transitional process is planned or unplanned, it is important to use the opportunity to help consolidate gains, review where things are, and leave the door open for the future. If a family feels that their experience with you has ended well, they will be more open to seeking help in the future, should it be needed. The process of moving on provides both the home visitor and the family a chance to put the experience into perspective, identify remaining concerns and challenges, and develop plans to help avoid future crises and problems.

SIDEBAR 7.1

Home Visitor and Family Tasks
During the Moving-on Phase

1. Mutually determine that it is time to begin a process of transition.
2. Set a time frame that includes the number of times you will see each other before saying goodbye.
3. Review what you have done together in the relationship:
   A. Evaluate your work together.
   B. Review and emphasize accomplishments—celebrate progress.
   C. Help the family see how the accomplishments can be applied to new situations.
   D. Explore your feelings and the family members' feelings about the changes that are about to occur in the relationship.
4. Establish a plan (the graduation, or moving-on plan).
   A. Talk about ways to prevent relapse.
   B. Identify supports and resources.
5. Establish an open door so the family feels comfortable asking for help in the future.
6. Say goodbye.

WHEN IS IT TIME TO THINK ABOUT MAKING A TRANSITION?

The decision to begin the process of transition that leads to graduation or moving on may come from either the home visitor or the family. Sometimes programs will have an established time limit, such as six months, two years, and so on. Alternatively some programs may permit a set number of visits and then expect the home visitor and the family to make other plans. Because many overburdened families need help experiencing continuity and are accustomed to experiences of loss and abandonment, it is important to clarify any time or visit restrictions from the beginning. Even so, many families, once they have settled into the relationship with the home visitor, will be reluctant to let go of it. The home visitor will need to keep these time constraints in mind and bring them into the family's awareness in plenty of time to allow for a process of transition.

Other situations that may cause the family to feel the relationship is ending too soon might involve circumstances in which the program loses its funding or the home visitor changes jobs. It is always a good idea to try to introduce these changes with enough time for you and the family to work through feelings and develop alternative plans.

There are times when the family does not feel engaged with the home visitor, or becomes frustrated with the process and disengages. In these cases the process of moving on may feel abrupt or premature to the home visitor. At times like these, you may find yourself feeling ineffective and trying to sell the program to the family. However, if the family has determined they are not interested in working with you, it is important to acknowledge this and work with the family to create as productive a closure as possible. In the future this experience of not being criticized or punished for leaving the program may make it easier for the family to seek help.

Early disengagement on the part of the family can be an important tool for self-reflection on the part of the home visitor, and can help you to improve your work with families. By finding out what you could have done to better engage the family, you can develop an understanding that will help you in the future. It is important during the moving-on process that you carefully listen to the family to help identify the barriers to engagement that might have occurred. Common barriers include such things as:

Attributes of the Home Visitor

Age, gender, race, religion, accent, and even height and weight can be barriers for some people. While it is not always possible to change these attributes, it is important to recognize them. Ideally the home visitor and the family can work through some of these attribution barriers by acknowledging them and examining their potential effects on developing a relationship. However, if the family is unable or unwilling to articulate these concerns or discuss them, they will probably end the relationship. If possible, find out if the family would like to be referred to someone else with less distracting attributes. Remember that your willingness to address these issues nonjudgmentally, while it may not keep the family on your caseload, may very well help the family later on. A fair and reasonable experience with you will promote an expectation that future contacts with helping professionals will be similar.

The Family Is Not Yet Ready to Commit to Change

Sometimes people need to test things out before making a commitment. Discomfort on the part of family members or mandates for services do not guarantee that the family is ready to engage in a change process. The home visitor needs to respect this and recognize the importance of leaving the family with a sense that the door is always open for future help. In chapter 3 we discussed the concept of readiness for change. If a family is ambivalent or not yet ready to commit, an experience that permits them to feel that they have been heard and treated with respect may help them to remain open to seeking help in the future.

Mistakes the Home Visitor Makes

We are all human, and sometimes, despite our best intentions, we may not listen, we may become impatient or judgmental, or in some other way alienate the family. When the family feels that they are not getting what they want and need, they may want to leave the relationship. Sometimes it is possible to work through these situations, but at other times the family may not be willing to continue. Again, use these opportunities to improve your work. By allowing the family to maintain a sense of control, and, in essence, to "fire" you from the relationship with them, you are enhancing their efficacy and allowing them to feel that they can take control of future helping relationships. While it is frustrating and painful to have a family leave prematurely because of something you have done or failed to do, it is important for both the home visitor and the family to understand what happened and learn from the experience. You may not always know when a mistake has been made. However, if the family stops coming to program activities or forgets home-visiting appointments, or in other ways avoids contact with you, it is worth exploring and following up in an open manner. The family may be relieved to be able to vent (even if you may feel that they are overreacting or using the situation as an excuse to disengage) without negative consequences. If you think of things from a broad time perspective, you may be able to see these early closures as steps along the family's path. Your willingness to allow them to maintain control may pay off in the future. While it is sometimes unpleasant to realize that you will not be the one to help the family, your willingness to behave professionally and therapeutically will enable a future helper to engage the family in a process of change.

In summary, it is time to initiate the process of transition in the relationship when goals have been reached, or when either the home visitor or the family has the need (for whatever reason) to disengage from the relationship. Regardless of the reasons for deciding to move on, it is important to try to complete the tasks of the moving-on phase of the relationship as much as possible.

Setting a Time Frame

Whether the transition is the result of program constraints, changes initiated by the home visitor, or changes initiated by the family, it is important to give yourself and the family time to work through some of your reactions and complete the transition so that there is a joint sense of closure. Of course, this is the ideal and there are times when the relationship ends abruptly without adequate processing. Try to let the family know from the beginning how and when the relationship will be undergoing a transition. For instance, if you are in a time-limited program, make sure at regular intervals to review this with the family. These reminders are a good time to review progress and change intervention goals.

At the end of the service period, or if you and the family have determined that the family's goals have been achieved, make a plan for transition. Explain the process to the family and work with them to determine how much time they will need to complete

SIDEBAR 7.2

Reactions to the Moving-on Process

There are may ways that the family and the home visitor may respond during this final phase of their work together. Reactions can be affected by the nature and quality of the relationship and the circumstances that led to the decision to move on. Personal experiences with loss and abandonment and other personal factors may influence both the family and the home visitor as they jointly negotiate the process of closing the current relationship and transitioning to something new. You will find yourself and the family experiencing some of the following reactions:

- Pride and a sense of accomplishment
- Hope and confidence for the future
- Denial
- Anger
- Sense of abandonment or loss—may lead to "I'll leave you right now so you can't leave me."
- Anxiety
- Relief
- Regression to old patterns
- Avoidance—finding new concerns, delaying the inevitable
- Wanting to be "friends"
- Sense of failure or incompetence
- Curiosity
- Guilt
- Frustration
- Satisfaction and a sense of competence

the steps identified in sidebar 7.1. If you acknowledge that you are in the final phases of the current service relationship and continue to focus with the family on the steps of transition, family members will gain a sense of control over the process, and they will be able to use the structure you establish to achieve closure. This step is very important for overburdened families, since so many of them have experienced unexplained or painful separations. For many families the idea of a process of saying goodbye will feel very strange and new. In this final stage of the relationship, you can model important relationship skills for the family.

If the relationship is changing prematurely, it is important to try to work through a closing process, even if it might be truncated. The home visitor can suggest to the family that a brief review of where things are along with an evaluation of what happened would be helpful. Be clear with yourself that in this circumstance you are not trying to win the family back, but instead are offering them a way to achieve closure and move on. This can be important because it reduces feelings of discomfort and failure and can help reinforce the family's sense that even though this relationship may not have worked out, there are still options open to them.

REVIEW WHAT YOU HAVE DONE TOGETHER

Review the work you and the family have shared. This will help the family integrate the experience and will reinforce the gains they have made. A review of where things were in the beginning, all of the experiences you and the family have shared, including frustrations and setbacks, will allow the family to both reinforce what they have learned and see themselves in a new light. During the review process, it is important to spend time exploring ways that the family's accomplishments can be applied to new situations.

An important component of the review process is an exploration of reactions to the transition. The home visitor and the family will experience many reactions to the changes in the relationship. Family members need to know that many of the things they are feeling are normal. This is a time when the home visitor may want to obtain consultation and support from colleagues, supervisors, or team members. It is always hard to say goodbye, and these transitional times present their own challenges and opportunities for both the family and the home visitor.

ESTABLISH A GRADUATION PLAN

One way to help the family take the step toward independence and separating from the relationship is to establish a graduation plan. The graduation plan includes a summary of accomplishments, reminders to help prevent relapses, and resources to help the family maintain their gains. The plan serves as a concrete reminder and reinforcer for the family. Sidebar 7.3 presents a format for a graduation plan, and sidebar 7.4 demonstrates how this format might be used with the Rodriguez family.

■

SIDEBAR 7.3

Family Graduation Plan

Family:

Home Visitor:

1. Review of achievements:

Family Member	Accomplishments	Plans to Maintain Accomplishments
A.		
B.		
C.		
D.		
E.		

2. Who will I/we call in an emergency?

3. Important phone numbers:

Doctor/health provider:

School(s):

Work:

Social service organizations/programs:

Police:

Other:

Congratulations

---■---

SIDEBAR 7.4

Family Graduation Plan

Family: Rodriguez

Home Visitor: Linda Wilson

1. Review of achievements:

Family Member	Accomplishments	Plans to Maintain Accomplishments
A. Sofia	1. Improved relationship with husband and son 2. Compliance with well baby visits 3. Improved household management and cleanliness 4. Completed GED and enrolled in community college	
B. Enrique	1. Improved English fluency 2. Enrolled in adult education and working on GED 3. Reduced drinking 4. Better relationship with wife and son 5. Increased relationship with family in Mexico	
C. Omar	1. Fewer infections and health problems 2. Improved attachment to parents 3. Development within normal range	

2. Who will I/we call in an emergency? Parenting for Healthy Children Help Line,

Mrs. Rodriguez, support group members (Olga)

3. Important phone numbers:

Parenting for Healthy Children: 619-777-7900

Mrs. Rodriguez: 011-664-132-3389

Support group (Olga): 619-768-4502

Doctor/health provider: Dr. Rios, 619-543-6498

School(s): Parenting for Healthy Children Play Group 619-777-7900

Work: (Enrique): Green Thumb Landscaping 619-630-2437

Social service organizations/programs: Parenting for Healthy Children Play Group,

Counseling at Briar Community College

Police:

Other:

Congratulations

Sometimes it is helpful to supplement the graduation plan with a summary describing the services provided, reasons for entering the program, results and follow-up. Sidebar 7.5 provides an example of such a summary, and sidebar 7.6 demonstrates the way that a termination summary might be prepared for the Rodriguez Family. This summary can be useful for quality management and as a way to help the family and the social worker wrap things up. It also serves as a useful starting point should the family return for additional services in the future.

ESTABLISH AN OPEN DOOR FOR THE FUTURE

Development and growth are lifelong processes. The family has worked with you intensively and accomplished goals that are important to them. However, this is the beginning, and not the end, of an exciting opportunity to grow and develop. Many times the overburdened family comes into a program at a point at which they are stuck. They may have given up on moving forward and may have been repetitively struggling with the same concerns and the same coping strategies. Family-support case management has helped to get things moving again. The family may be pleased with its progress, and perhaps even a little tired from the effort it has taken to get there. It is important to let family members know they are now engaged in an important growth process that does not stop here. Let them know that once they feel comfortable with their new coping skills and accomplishments they may find they want to venture into some new areas. This is normal and desirable. Help the family to recognize that asking for help again in the future is a sign of strength and continued growth. The home visitor at this stage has the opportunity to promote an attitude of openness to change and growth.

■

SIDEBAR 7.5

Case Termination Summary

Family:

Home Visitor:

I. Identifying Information and Reason for Services

Family members:

Marital status:

Presenting Problem:

II. Services Provided and Summary of Progress

III. Follow up

SIDEBAR 7.6

Case Termination Summary

Family: Rodriguez: Enrique, Sofia, Omar

Home Visitor: Linda Wilson

I. Identifying Information and Reason for Services

Family members:

Enrique, currently age 31, Latino male. Works as a foreman for a landscaping company. Born in Mexico. Legal residency

Sofia, currently age 27, Latina female, currently attending community college

Omar, currently 3 years, 8 months

Marital status: domestic partnership

Presenting Problem:

At the time of referral, Omar was exhibiting multiple infections, Parents were isolated and not familiar with child development. Poor social supports and evidence of insufficient parent-child attachment.

II. Services Provided and Summary of Progress

Linda Wilson was assigned as the home visitor. Team A managed the case. The family received home visiting and case management for three years, parenting groups and childcare for eighteen months. Sofia was seen by a therapist for a year. Omar is currently enrolled in our Early Success Play group and will be entering preschool in September.

The family has been receiving services for three years. Initially the parents were depressed, and social supports were weak. Baby was showing signs of poor health and insufficient attachment. Most of the work with this family focused on educating them about the child's needs, coaching them on how to better engage their son, and focusing on the individual development of each parent. Currently Sofia has completed her GED and is attending community college. She hopes to be a nurse's aide. Enrique has established legal residency and has steady employment as the foreman for a large landscaping company. He has been studying English and is beginning to work on his GED. Omar is developing within normal parameters. He attends playgroups and demonstrates normal emotional, social, and cognitive development. The couple has reached out to Enrique's family across the border and there are regular visits. Sofia attends a self-help parenting support group weekly.

Initial assessment information indicated concerns about insufficient social supports, parental depression, possible heavy drinking by Enrique, and lack of child development knowledge. The CES-D, MSS and AAPI were administered at the beginning of services and at the end. Scores on final administration indicated improved social supports, reduced depression, and improved parenting knowledge.

III. Follow up

This young family has improved its functioning considerably during the course of services. Both parents are committed to their son and have been able to recognize the importance of their own continued development and individuation to the well-being of their son. Enrique has developed a closer relationship with his family and this has increased the support system available to the family. Omar is doing well in the playgroup. The home visitor and the family have discussed the importance of both parents continuing with their current educational plans, and arrangements have been made to continue with Omar's preschool education. The family has developed a list of supports and emergency contacts and has agreed to contact the Parenting for Healthy Children Help Line if they feel overwhelmed. The home visitor, Linda Wilson, will call in six months to follow up.

SAYING GOODBYE

Once you and the family have reviewed progress, evaluated your work together, and established a plan for the future, it is time to bid each other farewell. This is not always easy. You have been working together intensely over a period of time and have gotten used to each other. Sometimes it is helpful to develop a goodbye ritual that allows you and the family to leave the relationship and yet retain it in memory. These rituals can be quite simple: a certificate of completion, a graduation ceremony, shared letters of farewell, or a small symbolic object can be used to signify the transition. You may want to develop a team or a program goodbye ritual. In this way you can let family members know well in advance what the transitional ceremony is. By using a similar ritual for all of the families you work with, you can avoid some of the boundary concerns that might emerge if each farewell were to be handled in an ad hoc fashion.

SUMMARY

This chapter discusses some of the considerations associated with ending the home-visiting relationship. The process of making a transition, whether to another home visitor, another program, or to graduation, requires a plan and some discussion of how gains will be maintained in the future. The importance of accomplishing a productive sense of closure is reviewed, and suggestions for managing the process are offered.

EIGHT

The Home Visitor as a Member of a Multidisciplinary Team

We have been examining how home visiting and case management can be used to help overburdened families to reduce potential adverse outcomes and improve life opportunities. These families have often had life experiences that increase their vulnerabilities. The home visitor can play a significant role in helping these families to enhance their resiliency. However, this is often more difficult than expected. The parents in overburdened families may have suffered from a variety of cumulative traumas and blows to their sense of self-efficacy. Long-standing mental health, attachment, and substance use issues may affect family relationships. There may be health and economic difficulties facing the family. While a home visitor with an organized approach to problem solving and case management can help the family, it is sometimes difficult for one person to have the skills and the training to effectively work with all dimensions of a family's situation.

Sometimes it is helpful to bring together a team of people with different, but complementary, skills in order to apply the most effective interventions with a family (Lewandowski and GlenMaye 2002). A typical team might include members with social work, mental health, child development, public health, and substance abuse expertise. Depending on the purposes of a given program, other members might include job coaches, probation and parole, and education, among others. This chapter will be of interest to home visitors, supervisors, and program administrators as we explore some of the ways that working in teams can be used in supporting vulnerable families.

WHY WORK IN TEAMS TO SUPPORT VULNERABLE FAMILIES?

Often the challenges facing families are personal, interactional, vocational, and economic. Community factors such as housing availability, educational and employment opportunities, community resources, and community cohesion can exert a powerful influence (Garbarino 1995; Carrilio 2001) Personal developmental challenges and coping styles as well as involvement with complex systems such as mental health, criminal justice, addictions treatment programs, health, education, and child welfare require helpers who understand both the clinical issues and the policy and program context in which these issues are expressed. By providing added expertise, multidisciplinary teams can be helpful in addressing the needs of vulnerable individuals and families (Carrilio, Cohen, and Goldman 1980; Carrilio and Eisenberg 1984; Stein and Santos 1998). Teams are often considered as a means of reducing burnout (Carrilio and Eisenberg 1984; Boyer and Bond 1999). Additionally teams can be useful in helping the family to maintain a sense of continuity (Carrilio 1998). The family is familiar with several team members; therefore, it is possible for the team to maintain a continued sense of caring and focus, even if a key team member, such as the home visitor, changes. Because many families struggle with stability and continuity, this aspect of working with teams can be helpful in providing the family with the security of knowing that even when changes occur in key personnel, such as the home visitor, the plan to which they have agreed, and the focus of service activities, will remain consistent. Another advantage to working in teams is the synergy of combined training

> ### SIDEBAR 8.1
>
> ## Why Work in Teams?
>
> - Makes more ideas/resources available for work with families—expands the possible choices of interventions
> - Balances the burden on individual team members
> - Helps team members to understand and balance their reactions to client families
> - Provides a forum for shared problem solving and ethical decision making on cases
> - Provides informal training and peer support
> - Promotes continuity of service for the client family
> - Promotes problem solving and worker efficacy
> - Reduces stress for team members
> - Encourages mutual accountability
> - Enhances communication and increases the efficiency of case management
> - Promotes quality management and efficient caseload management
> - Improved morale

and perspectives. Because the needs of vulnerable families can be so multilayered and complex, it is often helpful to utilize the experience, observations, and problem-solving skills of several people (Carrilio, Cohen, and Goldman 1980; Carrilio 2001).

Working in teams requires that the members of the team integrate their efforts. This is sometimes called Integrated Team Case Management (Carrilio 2001) because the whole team is jointly responsible for the families on its caseload. This shared case-management approach is in contrast to one in which a single home visitor is responsible for managing a caseload. In the integrated-team case-management approach, the home visitor is usually the key contact between the family and the team, but all members of the team manage the case collaboratively. The full resources of all team members, through case consultation and team supervision, are available to every family on the caseload. Members of the team come from different professional and experiential backgrounds, and are able to bring resources from their own networks into collaborative problem solving efforts with families.

Reasons for depending on the team as the source of intervention, rather than individual home visitors, no matter how well trained and skilled, include but are not limited to the following: 1) overburdened families can, in turn, easily overwhelm and overburden single workers; 2) countertransference issues are significant with these families, and the team approach helps to reduce these effects; 3) by using the specialists as a resource to the entire team, those team members with specific training and skills are not locked in to a single small caseload, but are able to utilize their skills on behalf of the entire caseload of the team; 4) because turnover is high among home visitors, helping families to connect with the team reduces disengagement when staff turnover occurs. Additionally, if a life span approach is taken, allowing families to reenter the program for "booster shots" at key periods of sensitivity, the relationship with the team is hypothesized as reducing barriers to reentry, since family members will not feel that strangers are handling them.

The case-management approach should focus upon an individualized family service plan, which is regularly reviewed and monitored by the team. No single service strategy is a stand-alone intervention. Services are embedded within a comprehensive and integrated service matrix, which is bound together through the case management and carried out by a multidisciplinary team. Case management involves more than simple linking, brokering, or referring to other services. The case-management function serves as the connecting process among the services utilized both within the team and from outside resources. It is dependent upon the development of a relationship between the team (usually through the home visitor) and the family.

HOW THE TEAM WORKS

The caseload belongs to the team and not to the individual worker. The family may develop a close relationship with a particular team member, often the home visitor. The home visitor utilizes the support of other team members, and, from time to time, other members of the team may be called upon to work closely with the client. Members of the team bring different educational, professional, and life experiences to their work with families. The team members provide training and consultation to each other on every case through team meetings, supervision, and formal training. Additionally all team members maintain an open door policy so their colleagues can consult with them informally throughout the day. The specialists serve as consultants, trainers, and standard setters in their respective areas, and are available to make home visits as an integral part of a family's overall plan. The home visitor makes use of these resources in developing a service plan, monitoring progress, and intervening when necessary. In the next chapter we will explore how home visitors and teams work together in programs that utilize psychoeducational groups as part of the overall program of family support.

TEAM MEETINGS

Team meetings are key to the effective functioning of the team as it provides support to overburdened families. Regular team meetings are essential. At these meetings the team discusses clinical concerns, case progress, administrative procedures, program development, logistics, solution strategies, and crisis management. During the team meeting, the team discusses its cases, clinical issues, quality management, policy and procedural issues, and provides support and education to team members. It is vital that every member of the team participates actively and regularly in team meetings, since this is where the team case management takes place. It is also important to make sure that enough time is allotted to cover all of the information needed by team members to carry on with their work. It is strongly suggested that team meetings occur at least once a week at a regularly scheduled time.

SUPERVISION

In addition to the group supervision that occurs in the team meetings, it is recommended that each team member receive regular individual supervision. During supervision, each case is reviewed and service plans are monitored and updated. By maintaining an open door policy, the team leader/supervisor assures that informal supervision is available during the periods

> SIDEBAR 8.2
>
> Structure of a Team Meeting
>
> • Discuss high priority cases/crises.
> • Discuss new families assigned to the team and identify lead staff.
> • Follow up on prior week's cases.
> • Review all cases.
> • Follow up on family service plans, new developments, assess current needs/risks/plan.
> • Update family plans as needed.
> • Review program procedures/policy questions, concerns, make administrative announcements.
> • Identify unmet client needs, training needs, program development issues.
> • Share data, progress, new resources.
> • Recognize accomplishments, progress, and successes.

between meetings. Home visitors and other team members are encouraged to review concerns or questions about cases at any time. Some teams place designated senior members on call during the evenings and weekends to provide guidance to home visitors if any of their assigned families experiences a crisis.

It is important for the team leader to clearly understand the relationship between the program's conceptual base and the goals and the objectives of service delivery. Supervision is most effective when the team leader is familiar with the conceptual model and is able to maintain consistency and flexibility within the model. The team leader guides the home visitor in developing an individualized approach to each family and helps the home visitor to establish and maintain appropriate boundaries with the families he/she serves. The team leader must also assure that all members of the team are working together and periodically take steps to intervene when personal or other barriers interfere.

The complexity of the home visitor's role and the scope of family needs make it imperative that there be adequate supportive supervision. It is important to assure that time be allocated for supervision and that this time is protected. Lack of supervision or poor supervision can lead to burnout and higher staff turnover as they feel unsupported and overburdened. Supervision in family-support programs is best carried out in a supportive, collaborative manner. Home visitors need a clear set of standards, training and assistance with the paperwork, and documentation requirements of the program. Documentation needs to be reviewed on a periodic basis; nevertheless, supervision that focuses on only the structural elements of the program is not sufficient to promote quality program delivery. There is a need for a special kind of collaborative

SIDEBAR 8.3

Supervision in a Family-Support
Home-Visiting Program

- Supportive supervision builds an atmosphere of respect, trust, openness, and mutual learning.
- Supervision maintains a sense of consistency and continuity.
- The team leader and home visitor are engaged in a mutual learning experience.
- Boundary issues in working with overburdened families are openly explored.
- The team leader empowers the home visitor by building problem-solving and assessment skills.
- The team leader acknowledges the stresses associated with working with overburdened families and helps the home visitor to contain his/her reactions by reframing and teaching.
- Supervision encourages self-observation and awareness of the way the home visitor's needs and concerns interact with the issues being raised in working with overburdened families.

communication in home-based program supervision that is based on a strong relationship with a supportive supervisor. The supervision experience should in many ways parallel a home visit process in that it is supportive, flexible, follows the lead of the supervisee, and provides new information in a way designed to increase self-confidence, flexibility, and empathy. If home visitors are expected to be respectful, thoughtful, and supportive during their home visits, to encourage discussion of problems, consideration of alternative points of view, and opportunities for reflection, it is essential that they be provided a similar experience during their own supervision. The home visitor who experiences respect and efficacy during supervision is more likely to reflect this in his/her work with families.

It is important for the home visitor and the supervisor to develop a relationship of trust. Consistency and regularly scheduled and kept appointments in supervision help to build trust and continuity in the relationship. Consistency also insures that supervision is a positive and preventive process rather than a venue to discuss only the crises or problems in home-visiting work. It also supports the home visitor in his/her efforts to provide consistency and continuity to families. Although team leaders/supervisors are often pulled in many directions because of their multiple responsibilities, it is essential to be consistently available for supervision and to avoid intrusions during the supervision time.

Supervision is a two-way process. The supervisor is responsible for creating an atmosphere that encourages collaborative supervision, and the home visitor must be ready to make good use of supervision. Here are a few suggestions:

- Understand what issues require your supervisor's input.
- Raise these issues in a timely manner. Do not wait or pretend the issue will fix itself.
- Utilize the supervisor's expertise; do not play the lone wolf.
- Listen to yourself (introspection); stay in touch with your feelings.
- Talk to your supervisor about any personal problems you are having that could be affecting your job performance.
- Initiate your own professional development and self-improvement; be proactive.
- Follow the chain of command; do not go behind someone's back.

■

Supervision Takes Many Forms

Individual supervision: Individual supervision is a basic ingredient for all home-based programs. The supervision should be regularly scheduled and appointments respected as a regular part of work responsibilities.

Group supervision: Group supervision is a way for team members to meet together to discuss cases and learn through this process. Group supervision is often effective in that issues raised in a case remind other home visitors of similar situations with their own caseload. In this way participation is often increased and a sense of safety and sharing of professional concerns is encouraged. A home visitor listening to a colleague present a case may develop new insights about his or her own work or may feel a greater degree of support and camaraderie. Group supervision can be a good addition to individual supervision, but should never replace it entirely, particularly since some of the group meetings are devoted to administrative purposes.

Peer support: Home visitors often help one another by listening, sharing resources, and providing new ideas. While this kind of activity should be encouraged and reflects a positive team approach, it is never sufficient in itself as a form of supervision.

Team member consultation and support: Team members possess different skills and training and are valuable resources. Part of the team leader/supervisor role is to help team members integrate their knowledge into the complex home-visiting process.

Crisis supervision: All home visitors must have access to their supervisor in times of crisis and in situations where they need assistance immediately, for example, in a situation where they have witnessed a potentially abusive situation, a suicidal parent, or criminal behavior.

Ongoing availability: In reality a great deal of supervision happens informally in hallways, offices, and on the phone. Although this kind of availability is important and often essential in terms of a crisis or an upsetting situation, it does not and should never be expected to replace regular scheduled supervision time.

THE CHALLENGE OF WORKING ON A TEAM

Being a team member is a challenge and is not always as easy as it sounds. While the team can serve an important role in helping family-support home visitors to identify needs and resources, maintain morale, set and maintain boundaries with families, and avoid becoming overburdened themselves, the team has its own dynamics, and is, in fact, a group. Every member of the team is called upon regularly to maintain team spirit and effectiveness. Sometimes this is difficult because team members disagree, compete, experience burnout, or bring personal issues into the group process. This is normal when people get together in groups. Every member of the team needs to work to develop and maintain a cohesive, functioning team.

There is not clear evidence that working in teams is any more effective than a home visitor working on his or her own (Rapp and Goscha 2004; Carrilio, Cohen, and Goldman 1980). However, in order to be effective, it is clear that both teams and individual home visitors require the support and guidance of a seasoned professional. It is therefore quite important to assure that home visitors receive supervision and that whether in a team or through a well-experienced professional supervisor, home visitors are helped to identify and manage the complex, multifaceted needs of highly vulnerable families.

It is important to understand what factors contribute to team effectiveness and what can contribute to less-than-effective team functioning. The supervisor and all team members need to attend to team dynamics in an active way. A key part of effective teamwork is a sense of clear, agreed-upon purpose and mutual respect (Lewandowski and GlenMaye 2002).

SIDEBAR 8.5

What Is Expected of the Supervisor

- Evaluate staff on a regular basis to ensure quality of services:
  - Formally, using administrative personnel procedures.
  - Informally, during individual supervision.
- Provide training on issues faced by home visitors.
- Get input from all the team members on training needs.
- Utilize team specialists whenever possible (delegate).
- Allow the home visitor time off to attend conferences, seminars, and workshops.
- Host community professionals to provide in-service training.
- Create a culture of trust, rapport, safety, and professionalism.
- Staff retreats: Ask the staff what **they** want to do.
- Rewards and recognition: Can be as small as a post-it note saying, "Great job!"
- Clear guidelines and procedures; consistency.
- Limit gossip among staff: Share information willingly, and timely; avoid the rumor mill.

SIDEBAR 8.6

What Is Expected of the Home Visitor

- Understand what issues require your supervisor's input.
- Raise these issues in a timely manner: Do not wait or pretend the issue will fix itself.
- Utilize supervisor's expertise: Do not play the lone wolf.
- Be specific; getting to the point saves time and energy.
- Use self-awareness regarding personal problems and countertransference issues.
- Listen to yourself (introspection); stay in touch with your feelings.
- Talk to your supervisor about any personal problems you are having that could be affecting your job performance.
- Initiate your own professional development and self-improvement; be proactive.
- Offer suggestions for trainings.
- Look for training opportunities and talk to your supervisor about attending.
- Utilize the team specialists' wealth of expertise and experience.
- Follow the chain of command; no going behind someone's back.
- Keep lines of communication open with team members.
- Be considerate of team members' time constraints.
- Listen closely to feedback from team members; think about what will work.

SUMMARY

This chapter explores the ways in which family home visitors function on family-support teams. While not every program will utilize a team approach, the use of teams is common in family-support contexts, primarily because teams can contribute to effectively addressing the multiple and complex needs of families. It can be challenging to work on a team, and being a team member requires that all members of the team share a sense of purpose and establish mutual respect. Teams provide an arena for support, problem solving, and supervision. Effectively functioning teams can enhance the ability of individual home visitors to work effectively with families.

SIDEBAR 8.7

Characteristics of an Effective Team

- Interdependence
- Open and honest communication
- Continuous quality improvement
- Shared goals
- Learning environment
- Shared power and control
- Respect for differences
- Trust and openness
- Decision making by consensus
- Sense of belonging

SIDEBAR 8.8

Why Teams Sometimes Do Not Work Effectively

- Different expectations of self, team members, client families
- Different ideas about how to intervene
- Concerns about status and authority
- Personality styles affect group dynamics
- Experience and skills in dealing with conflict
- Experience and skills in consensus building
- Different ideas about sharing power and control
- Unresolved personal issues and needs
- Reluctance to develop trust
- Fear of taking risks

NINE

Integrated-Team Case Management

While home visiting is the centerpiece of the integrated-team case-management approach, many programs encourage families to apply what they learn in a supportive environment at the program offices. This is often called a center-based service component. Commonly this means attending groups and organized activities with other families who are also involved in the program. In addition to giving members of the team a chance to interact with and observe families in a community context, groups give families a chance to practice new skills in a safe environment and to begin to move out of the isolation that many of these families experience. Social isolation is a significant problem in these families, not only because it creates stress in and of itself, but also because without the input of others, parents may make poor decisions in managing their daily activities. This chapter will be of use to home visitors who are working in programs that include parent education and other groups. Supervisors and administrators may find some guidance for the development of a group psychoeducational component in the discussion that follows.

An approach that has worked well in many home-visiting programs consists of a structured group for the parents paralleled by age-appropriate groups for the children (Yoshikowa 1995; Carrilio 1998; Carrilio 2001). Parenting education and support groups have been successfully utilized to improve the parent's understanding of their child and to offer opportunities to practice and learn new skills (Cowen 2001; Carrilio 2001; MacDonald and Sayger, 1998). The group component of the program provides the team with a way to observe the parents and children outside of the home setting to get a sense of how they get along with others, how the children are doing with peers, and how well they are integrating the work they are doing with the home visitor. Observations in the group setting permit the home visitor to follow up in a highly individualized way with the family and to more specifically tailor interventions to meet the family's needs. The center-based environment can also serve as a nonthreatening way for families to meet other team members.

When coordinated with, and reinforced by, home-visiting case management, these psychoeducational skill-building groups can be extremely powerful. The goal is twofold: to assist parents to consolidate their newly acquired parenting skills and to promote the reduction of debilitating isolation. New ideas about issues that are relevant to the families in their day-to-day lives can be learned and shared in a group setting and supported at home during regular meetings with the home visitor. In the group parents have an opportunity to experience the support and empathy of other parents who have been (or are) in similar situations. This may be the first time they have had the experience of being listened to, validated, or supported in any of their parenting concerns.

A primary benefit of the group component of a comprehensive family-support program is the reduction in the family's sense of isolation. The risk to families already experiencing stress, who lack appropriate supports and resources to deal with that stress, is increased dramatically by isolation. The experience of isolation can contribute to parent involvement in drug/alcohol abuse, domestic violence, child maltreatment, and other harmful behavior. Being out in the world in an environment which is safe, structured, consistent, and positive, provides overburdened parents and their children with a corrective experience. Emotional growth and reparation occur in an environment which is supportive and safe and which addresses the day-to-day concerns of importance to the parent.

Group facilitators and staff members who are available to group members before, during, and after the group do a great deal of modeling. Parents are patiently guided through the process each week, revisiting the rules and reinforcing their accomplishments. Parents are consistently encouraged to believe in themselves and are rewarded when they accomplish their goals, even if those goals are as mundane as coming to the group on a weekly basis without absences.

Another benefit to the group component of the model is that it is often a good way to involve fathers. It is suggested that at least some of the groups be in the evening, and that the groups be culturally and linguistically appropriate to the population being served. Evening groups encourage fathers to come and they also give the mothers the message that they can go to work or school and still participate fully in the program.

STRUCTURAL COMPONENTS OF THE CENTER-BASED GROUP SERVICES

Center-based groups provide an opportunity for families to interact with other members of the team. Staff with training in psychoeducational groups and child development have an opportunity to work with family members through structured groups. There are seven key structural components to the suggested center-based component of an integrated-team case-management program:

1. Structured parent skill-building and support groups led by one or more members of the case-management team
2. Age-appropriate children's groups coordinated with the parenting skill groups
3. Interactive groups with parents and very young children
4. Childcare
5. Transportation that is incorporated into the family service plan
6. Staff debriefing and problem-solving case coordination after each group session

7. Utilization of "graduates" and family members who have been in the program to mentor and provide peer support to newer members

1. Structured Parent Skill Building and Support Groups

Many overburdened families have attended parenting classes in the past. Most of these classes have excellent curricula and provide good common sense information on a variety of family topics. However, many overburdened families have difficulty translating what they have learned in these classes into day-to-day life in their own homes. Some family-support home-visiting programs have developed an integrated series of highly structured parent groups which incorporate teaching and experiential elements and focus very heavily on helping parents to integrate the material they learn. Every aspect of the group process, including transportation and signing in, and the details of group operation are carefully geared toward teaching and providing parents with a structured environment to practice new skills.

2. Age-Appropriate Children's Groups Coordinated with the Parenting Skill Groups

Age-appropriate groups for the children, teaching them important social skills and helping them learn to respond to the new skills their parents are learning, play an important role in helping families to break out of a spiral of helplessness and poor relating. Children learn how to identify and express their needs, work cooperatively with others, handle stress and anger, and develop self-regulation skills.

3. Interactive Groups with Parents and Young Children

Younger children and their parents are invited to attend interactive parenting groups in which they observe other parents with their infants and young children and receive coaching on ways to interact with their own child. Here the parents can observe other children and receive practical hints about how to enhance their child's development. For many overburdened parents, who themselves were poorly nurtured, it is necessary to actually teach them to tune into their children and to play with their children. The entire family is encouraged to attend in order to learn together.

4. Childcare

Many of the families who most benefit from family-support programs cannot afford childcare, and many of them make poor decisions about childcare. In order to assure that the children are safe while their parents are in groups, many family-support home-visiting programs offer childcare. An additional benefit of providing childcare is that the staff has an opportunity to observe the children and identify concerns for the home visitor to follow up on if necessary.

5. Transportation

Because many overburdened families have significant transportation barriers, transportation to groups and other center-based activities is an important component in the early part of the home-visiting and family-support relationship. However, a careful balance between dependence and autonomy needs to be managed, and families are encouraged as part of their work with the program to begin identifying alternatives and developing plans to get themselves to the center-based activities. Working through transportation plans can be an excellent way to work in a protected setting with the families on planning, problem solving, and other skills which will help them not only in their parenting, but in other important areas of their daily lives.

6. Staff Debriefing and Problem-Solving Case Coordination after Each Group Session

Members of the team staff all of the group components listed above. Frequently there are logistical, procedural, and clinical issues that come up each session. It is suggested that all of the staff who have been part of a particular group session meet briefly afterward to discuss important issues and concerns which have come up as a result of observations and events in the groups. This is a time for problem solving, identification of concerns, and notation of progress. All of the staff working in the combined components of a group session serve as a mini-team. The staff assess how families are doing and provide information to each other and to the larger team. The combined observations of all staff, working with the family, helps the team to monitor case progress, and to determine whether the service plan needs to be reviewed.

7. Utilization of "Graduates" and Family Members Who Have Been in the Program to Mentor and Provide Peer Support to Newer Members

Many of the group components build upon concepts of psychosocial rehabilitation, which focuses on developing efficacy and life skills through a psychoeducational process which breaks learning down into small, manageable pieces that can be mastered at the family's own pace (Carrilio 1998). At every step of the program, family members are encouraged to develop and use new skills and to practice these skills in the safety of the center environment. Whenever possible, families should be encouraged to progressively take on tasks associated with registration, orientation, supporting new members, and problem solving during center-based activities. This gives families a chance to experience efficacy and to practice what they are learning in a setting that provides support.

It is recommended that each site develop a plan for participants to incrementally become involved with helping with center-based activities and mentoring of new families. Ideally some family members can move through progressive stages that will enable them to retain their supportive connection to staff at the same time that they develop more and more autonomy. Some programs may want to establish strategies for allowing selected graduates to join the staff as they move through progressive stages of responsibility and development. The group program and the incorporation of family involvement in the operation of the program allows the program to continue providing a "holding" function for families at the same time that it encourages the development of new skills.

SOME GUIDELINES FOR SETTING UP GROUPS

Logistics

It is recommended that at least some of the groups be held in the evening or on weekends in order to accommodate parents who work or go to school. This is also an excellent way to increase the involvement of fathers, grandfathers, and partners. Room availability, staffing, and other factors may affect individual program decisions about group times, but once set, the time should be adhered to firmly. Clear rules regarding attendance, lateness, and absences need to be established and maintained with consistency.

As soon as the initial contact or request for group is made, a registration packet should be sent to the parent describing the fundamental group rules and structure. In some programs the home visitor brings the registration materials to the family and works with them to prepare it. The registration packet includes the forms for registering in the group. The information in the packet explains basic procedures to the parents with respect to transportation, expectations of the group, roles, and policy issues such as not bringing sick children into the center. The registration packet shows the parent that there is an organized structure, and this helps to bind and reduce anxiety, set expectations, and establish the clear, consistent, firm limits that will build an experience of safety and predictability for families attending the groups.

Rules of Conduct

Parents and children need to know clearly what behaviors will and will not be tolerated. There need to be clearly spelled-out expectations so the parents know how to access transportation, handle arrival and childcare, and how to pick up their children after the group. The home visitor and team work with the parent to assure that the family is ready to engage at each group session. This includes such seemingly simple things as having the children fed and dressed and planning for transportation to get to the group on time. For some families these logistical skills are extremely challenging and will require considerable support. Assisting the parents by increasing their awareness and efficacy in day-to-day tasks can be both therapeutic and empowering. Mastering developmental tasks through the reinforcement of role definition and practice opportunities provides an emotional framework that the parents can use in many areas of their lives.

The management of logistical expectations serves both to maintain the safety of all participants and staff and to provide "grist for the mill." The families' struggles with managing these expectations are likely to take up large amounts of time. These apparently endless struggles with behavior management, boundaries, and limits should not be seen as a waste of time, but rather as opportunities to work with the families to help them experience success and efficacy. Team members need to be comfortable with setting limits firmly, but not rigidly. Families are building important skills just by coming to the group and responding to the group structure.

Each piece of the group is highly structured in the hope of addressing the lack of regularity and stability in the lives of overburdened families. For example, if transportation to group is provided, it is a good idea to provide a window in which families must sign up for transportation. The parent would be responsible to notify the program by a specified time if they will need transportation that week. This process may prove to be very challenging for many families. However, consistently working with parents to master these tasks provides them with a successful experience they can begin to integrate into a growing repertoire of coping and adaptive skills. As basic as this example appears, it actually represents a very solid accomplishment that the parent can utilize in other situations. It is the mastery of a developmental task that promotes the advancement to a level of higher functioning.

The group fosters a step-by-step method of growth for the families that assists them in compensating for some of their own deprived childhood experiences which may have significantly impaired their adaptive functioning. The group attempts to provide the parents with structure and consistency that they may have craved as children, but never experienced.

QUALITY MANAGEMENT

The quality management component of groups involves weekly debriefing sessions and regular meetings among the staff engaged in providing center-based activities. An integrated parent and parent-child curriculum needs to be developed and reviewed/revised regularly. Center-based groups are constantly refreshed and revitalized by exploring as a team the activities which worked, and those that need to be changed, improved, or discarded. In this way the center-based program remains lively, fresh, and new. The multidisciplinary team, the families, and the center-based services staff are encouraged to feel ownership of the center-based group program and to be constantly seeking ways to improve and enliven program activities.

It is recommended that programs research existing parenting curricula and choose one or more of these curricula for use in the center-based component of the program. In developing and scheduling sessions, it is important to pay attention to the *process* of how the center-based component is delivered. The groups are intended to provide a safe, consistent environment that enhances learning by offering both parents and children structured opportunities to practice and to integrate the skills they learn. Curriculum materials serve as a starting place for a center-based program, but each program will need to tailor the modules to their own strengths and to client needs.

In applying any curriculum it is important to assure that the didactic portion of the curriculum does not become overwhelming, and the implementation is consistent with the program approach and model. Additionally the team needs to work together to assure that the curriculum is delivered in a manner that is consistent with the needs and characteristics of the clients being served. In short the way in which the curriculum is built into the program is at least equally important as the specific didactic material presented.

SIDEBAR 9.1

The Rodriguez Family: Parenting Classes

Enrique and Sofia began attending classes sporadically at about the same time they began accepting visits from the home visitor. Omar, their son, began coming to the child development groups that run concurrently with the parenting classes when he was nine months old.

Initially Sofia would leave the group frequently to check on Omar, who in turn, would cry as Sofia tried to leave the room. Sofia would rock Omar mechanically and push his bottle at him. She seemed to want to show that she was a good mother, but was not able to differentiate Omar's signals, thereby appearing unresponsive and wooden to the staff running the groups. Staff worked with Sofia to help her focus more on specific messages from Omar, and they provided her with information about attachment and stranger anxiety. Once Sofia recognized that his protests were normal, she became less anxious and self-critical about leaving Omar during the groups. After about six weeks of one-on-one coaching and support to Sofia for separating from Omar for the ninety minute parenting group, both Sofia and Omar were able to tolerate the separation. Staff noted that Omar seemed less anxious and more relaxed as Sofia began to feel comfortable that he was behaving like a normal baby.

In the group Enrique was silent and withdrawn, especially when Sofia was in the children's room with Omar. In response to questions about parenting expectations, Enrique would indicate that while his child was young he did not think he had much of a role, and he was leaving the care taking to Sofia. Enrique often indicated that "men don't change diapers" or soothe crying babies. He expressed concern that his son would be a sissy because of his mother's pampering every time he cries.

After Enrique and Sofia settled into the group routine, they attended regularly, although it was several months before they began engaging in conversations during the group. Both Enrique and Sofia presented as quiet and shy during the mingling before class and during the break. After they had been coming for about six months, the couple began to sit near another young couple and talking quietly with the couple before the group and during breaks. It was at this point that Enrique began to volunteer opinions and ask questions in the group. After a few weeks of this, Sofia, too, began to be more involved in group discussions. Sofia told the home visitor that she felt comfortable in the group and very much enjoyed the group routines and rituals. Being able to count on knowing what would happen helped her to feel comfortable. Enrique found that hearing how other people were doing things was helpful, and he felt relieved to know that other people struggled with some of the same questions and concerns he had.

The home visitor and group facilitator met periodically to review the family's progress and to assure that the group and home-visiting interventions were well integrated. At six-month intervals the group facilitator administered the AAPI to identify any improvements in parenting knowledge.

Enrique and Sofia attended parenting groups for eighteen months. Their AAPI scores at the end of the eighteen months indicated improvements on all dimensions, although both the home visitor and Sofia recognized that Sofia would need more coaching on how to respond empathically to Omar, who at this point was an active two year old. Sofia and her home visitor recognized that one of Sofia's barriers had to do with her own weak sense of self and as the group experience was ending, Sofia decided to seek individual counseling. Enrique's scores indicated a more realistic understanding of Omar's developmental capacities, and Enrique indicated a willingness to consider alternatives to corporal punishment. Even though at the end of the groups Omar was a typically grandiose two year old, Enrique was able to put this into perspective and recognize that some of Omar's apparent defiance was a normal and healthy part of development.

SUMMARY

In this chapter we have explored some of the ways in which parent education and other developmentally focused groups can be used in conjunction with family-support home visiting. Groups can be helpful in reducing isolation, offering concrete information and skills, and providing structured opportunities for practicing new skills. In some programs the use of groups may allow for a system that allows successful program participants to move into helping roles. Groups, like home visiting, need to be carried out in a way that reflects the program's conceptual model. For this reason, in planning concrete issues, such as time, facilities, curriculum, registration, and group policies, it is important to assure that decisions are consistent with the program model.

TEN

The Home Visitor's Role in Quality Management and Evaluation

Frequently home visitors are uncertain about the paperwork in a program. Many times the forms and written requirements seem like a diversion from the real work of helping families. Home visitors often report feeling resentful and overburdened themselves by the mountain of paperwork they are required to complete. Sometimes home visitors feel like the paperwork is a way to check up on them. Many home visitors feel they are good with people and they should not be asked to use their time filling out forms and writing notes. While these are very honest and understandable reactions, it is useful to think in a different way about the question of monitoring and evaluating one's work. This chapter is intended to help home visitors better understand how paperwork is part of the job and to help them see these recording tasks as less onerous. For supervisors and program directors, this chapter may provide some ideas about how to structure documentation requirements and organize data collection systems.

Figure 10.1 Quality management and evaluation

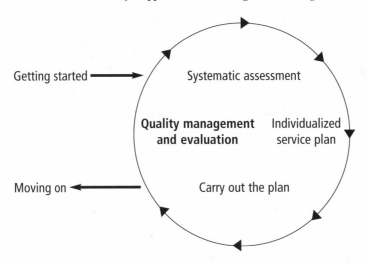

Family-Support Home-Visiting Case-Management Process

Monitoring consists of keeping track of what you are doing, self-reflection, checking in with the family, and evaluating both quality and progress on an ongoing basis. This sounds like a lot, and you may be wondering why the home visitor should be paying attention to these things. After all, your job is to engage families and maintain a supportive, therapeutic relationship with them. All of this focus on forms, data, and measuring outcomes is a waste of time. Or is it?

HOW DO WE MONITOR AND EVALUATE PROGRAMS?

Monitoring means that we are keeping track of what we are doing. Good practice requires that the home visitor keep records to help organize the case-management

---

■

SIDEBAR 10.1

Why Monitor and Evaluate Programs?

- Did we do what we said we would do?
- Did we do it well?
- Were services provided effectively? Efficiently?
- Did we get the results we expected?
- Are families doing better as a result of participating in services?
- Which services were effective? Which were not?
- Are the program results worth the cost and investment?

---

work. It is important to use records to remind yourself of where things are with the family, and to provide information so that if a team member or your supervisor needs to become involved in your absence, they will have enough information to provide the appropriate interventions. There are two things the home visitor needs to monitor: 1) process and 2) outcomes. Process monitoring captures information about what happened, such as how many visits you have had, how long you were with the family, what services you provided. Outcomes monitoring tries to find out if the family has improved and if your work has had an impact.

Process monitoring helps to assure you are carrying out the expected program activities given the logic model your program is based upon. For example, if you are part of a program that follows a model of weekly one hour home visits focused on child development and family relationships, you would use process data to check yourself and see if, in fact, your visits with families were taking place weekly, for one hour, and focusing on the specified content. Process data tells you what you did and allows you to compare what actually happened in the program to what was supposed to happen, based on the program model. Usually no home visitor can carry out the suggested program approach perfectly, but the process data will give you, your team, and your supervisor a good idea of how close or how far your actual activities come to meeting the ideal. When there are discrepancies between what you thought you were doing and what the process data says you are doing, it is important to view this as an opportunity to both improve your own work and perhaps identify things in the program that need to be changed. Home visitors are sometimes concerned about using process data to evaluate performance because they fear retribution or they think that it makes them look incompetent. However, by using the information to understand what is going on in the program and identifying possible changes in policy, procedures, or training that are needed, the data can be used to help you do a better job.

The idea of measuring outcomes is often a little frightening to home visitors, and even their supervisors and administrators. Outcomes tell us whether, even if we have

SIDEBAR 10.2

Monitoring Process and Quality

1. What are the program expectations?
   A. Number of visits
   B. Time to spend with families
   C. Frequency of visits
   D. Activities to be performed by the home visitor
2. Are the activities required by the program happening?
3. Is the family meeting its goals?
4. Have you identified barriers in the program or the resource system that make it hard to work with families?
5. Are you carrying out the plan you and the family agreed to?
6. Are there changes in your work or in the program that would improve effectiveness?
7. Are you seeing any results in the outcome measures that the program uses?
8. If improvements were suggested in the past, have they been implemented?
9. Have these changes made a difference?

performed the program perfectly, our work has had any effect. It is possible to have process data that reflects what is called model fidelity (adherence to the suggested elements of the program model) and yet does not show any outcomes (Chaffin, Bonner, and Hill 2001). Home visitors and the programs they work for are often concerned that if their work appears to be ineffective, the funding for the program will be cut. Depending on the funding source and program context, this can seem more or less a threat (Carrilio 2006). Nevertheless, the question needs to be asked: "Did the services and approach suggested by this program have an impact on the issue we were trying to affect?" If the answer is "no," it is important to recognize that this does not mean that the staff did not do their jobs or that they are not skilled case managers. What it does mean is that the way the program is structured, or the specific components of the program, are not addressing the identified concerns sufficiently. This information needs to be studied carefully by program staff at all levels, as well as by evaluators, administrators, and funders, to determine what changes might improve program effectiveness.

Most programs monitor process data because it helps to manage caseloads and often provides funders with information about who is being served, what is being provided, and how often. Basic demographic information that provides a description of the population receiving program services is often part of process data collection. Home visitors are familiar with forms that ask for the name, address, education, and other descriptive information about the families they work with. Home visitors sometimes resent having to write down everything they do. Depending on how easy it is to record this basic process data, home visitors may vary considerably in the accuracy and consistency with which they document basic process information.

Documenting your work is important. Some version of the tools suggested in Sidebar 10.3 is usually part of most program procedures. Make sure that you understand what is expected of you with respect to case documentation in your program. All programs utilize some form of case record system. Likewise, many programs use a manual or computerized client data system to gather essential process data on service activities. In the area of outcomes, programs vary considerably. Some programs will be satisfied with only conducting process recording. However, more and more, the organizations and people who fund human services programs are demanding that programs demonstrate effectiveness and measure outcomes (Kettner, Moroney, and Martin 1999; Lewis et al. 2001).

FAMILY CASE RECORDS

The case record is a folder that contains all of the relevant details about individual families with whom you work. The forms and information in the case record depend upon the requirements of the program and its funders. A case record helps you to communicate with your supervisor and team and offers a quick reference when you are making referrals or trying to keep track of your activities with a family.

Every program has its own unique forms and ways of collecting the important information in a case record. Sidebar 10.4 describes the key components of any case record. Your program may call these components by different names, but if you review the files on your caseload, you will most likely see these components in one form or another.

Referral/Intake Form

This form is used to collect initial information and often serves to register a family in the program. The information may be provided by the family or by another agency or professional referring the family to your program. The information on this form usually contains contact information, a brief description of the reason the family has been referred, and perhaps some basic demographic information if it is relevant, such as age, marital status, and living situation. In many programs, the intake/referral form is used to initiate the program's services.

Consent, Confidentiality, Clients' Rights Forms

The case record should clearly document that the family is aware of their rights and that family members understand the program's confidentiality procedures. It is important for the family to understand the services they will be receiving and to provide written consent to share relevant information with specific professionals, systems, and individuals. Early in your contact with the family it is important to review confidentiality and its limits. The family should be made aware of mandated reporting requirements. Many programs ask families to sign something indicating they have been informed of the confidentiality procedures and understand them. If there is a need to obtain or share information with doctors, schools, the courts, or other outside individuals, it is necessary for you to obtain written consent. This consent should be very specific and detail exactly what can and cannot be shared with others.

Assessment Narrative and Summary

The case record should contain an analysis and summary of all of the data you collect during the assessment process. A detailed discussion of the assessment process is contained in chapter 4. If your agency uses standardized screening and assessment tools, these should be included in the case record. Placing these data in one place makes it easier for you and other team members to find and review information during case planning and periodic reviews. The assessment narrative pulls everything together and gives a good overall picture of the family and their current needs, strengths, and challenges (see sidebar 4.7 for an example of an assessment summary).

Family Service Plan

The individualized family service plan described in chapter 5 is a key part of the case record. Programs develop their own formats for these plans, but they often contain the elements described in sidebar 5.2. The plan is a way to summarize the family's goals and the specific action plan you have developed with them. The service plan is what organizes your work with the family, and it should be reviewed at regular intervals. The updated plans that result from these regular reviews also belong in the case record. Many programs establish procedures for plan reviews as part of an overall plan for quality management.

Specialized Plans

In chapter 5 we explored the use of specialized plans for crisis management, establishing family safety, and other purposes requiring detailed attention. If you and the family have developed a specialized plan, it should be included in the case file and updated periodically.

Progress Notes

Progress notes are a key part of the case record. They provide succinct information about what is going on with the family, and what you have done recently. It is important to keep progress notes up to date so your supervisor or other team members can pick up where you left off should this be necessary. The progress notes are also a good way to help you remember what is going on with each of the families with whom you are working. Ideally progress notes provide the narrative for items contained in client information systems data.

———————————————————◼———————————————————

Tips for Writing Good Progress Notes

1. Remember: Progress notes are a good way for you and your supervisor to keep track of the work you are doing with families.
2. Include all of the information another home visitor would need to know if he/she suddenly had to work with this family for any reason.
3. Stay focused on the family's goals and service plan.
4. Do not make interpretations or conclusions— just describe what you observe.

The progress note should be brief, clear, and descriptive. In a brief paragraph, describe:

Date of contact

Which family members you saw or spoke with (eg., *I met with Mrs. Brown, Tanisha, 8, and Frederick, 3.*)

The significant topics you covered (e.g., *We reviewed the service plan and made sure we had each done our agreed upon tasks for this week. Mrs. Brown indicated that she did not call the job counselor because she was too down. I asked her about what "being down" meant and wondered if she would be able to make the call this coming week. She said she would try. I told her that since she was so down, it might be a good idea to consider meeting with our doctor to see if her depression was returning. She agreed and asked me to make an appointment. I called the office from the Brown home and made an appointment for next Tuesday at 9 A.M. We discussed logistics of getting to the appointment.*)

Any concerns. These should be described very specifically (e.g., *Mrs. Brown appeared unusually tired at our meeting. She yelled frequently at Tanisha, who became angry in turn and broke a toy. Frederick appeared detached from his*

mother and sister. Mrs. Brown may need to be evaluated for depression and possible medications.)

Observations of progress (e.g., *Mrs. Brown appears to have reached a plateau. She has not called the job counselor, which is part of the plan. She is getting angry with Tanisha and ignoring Fredrick. We have agreed to an evaluation for depression.*)

Summary of action steps (e.g., *Mrs. Brown agreed to call the job counselor and to attend an evaluation session with the program psychiatrist next Tuesday at 9 A.M. I agreed to call her one hour before her appointment to remind her and to talk about any problems she might be having with getting to the appointment.*)

When will you meet next? (e.g., *We agreed to meet on Wednesday, after the meeting with the psychiatrist so we can go over things.*)

Here is the completed progress note for this visit with Mrs. Brown and her children:

January 6:
I met with Mrs. Brown, Tanisha, 8, and Frederick, 3. We reviewed the service plan and made sure that we had each done our agreed upon tasks for this week. Mrs. Brown indicated that she did not call the job counselor because she was too down. I asked her about what "being down" meant and wondered if she would be able to make the call this coming week. She said she would try. I told her that since she was so down, it might be a good idea to consider meeting with our doctor to see if her depression was returning. She agreed and asked me to make an appointment. I called the office from the Brown home and made an appointment for next Tuesday at 9 A.M. We discussed logistics of getting to the appointment.

Mrs. Brown appeared unusually tired at our meeting. She yelled frequently at Tanisha, who became angry in turn and broke a toy. Frederick appeared detached from his mother and sister. Mrs. Brown may need to be evaluated for depression and possible medications. Mrs. Brown appears to have reached a plateau. She has not called the job counselor, which is part of the plan. She is getting angry with Tanisha and ignoring Frederick. We have agreed to an evaluation for depression. Mrs. Brown agreed to call the job counselor and to attend an evaluation session with the program psychiatrist next Tuesday at 9 A.M. I agreed to call her one hour before her appointment to remind her and to talk about any problems she might be having with getting to the appointment. We agreed to meet on Wednesday, after the meeting with the psychiatrist so we can go over things.

Service Tracking Forms

Many programs develop a method, either manual, or computerized, to keep track of the services you provide. These data can be used for reports, quality management, and case planning. If your agency uses forms to record your work with families, these forms should be included in the case record.

Graduation Plan

In chapter 7 we reviewed the process of moving on and transitioning to new relationships, and suggested that you leave the family with a graduation plan they can use to continue their progress. This plan should be included in the case record. Sidebar 7.3 offers an example of a family graduation plan. Should the family return, or need assistance in the future, the graduation plan serves as a good starting point for reengagement. The graduation plan can also be a useful part of quality management and evaluation activities.

Transition/Graduation Summary

The graduation summary reviews the case and concisely describes what the initial situation was, what was done, and where things stand at the point at which the family is transitioning out of services. The transition/graduation summary helps you to get an overview of the entire relationship with the family and can be a useful tool if the family returns to the program at a later date. Sidebar 7.4 provides an example of a graduation summary.

MANAGEMENT INFORMATION SYSTEMS

Many home-visiting and case-management programs utilize some form of management information system to capture data on what is happening in the program. These information systems primarily collect and process data, that is, who did what, with whom, where, how long, and how often. Some information systems are able to capture rudimentary trend and outcomes data by using standardized measures and entering these data into the information system. Frequently home visitors (and their supervisors) are not comfortable with these systems (Carrilio 2005a; Carrilio, Packard, and Clapp 2003), especially if they are computerized. However, it is important to recognize that collecting data on what you are doing can be extremely helpful in maintaining high quality programs.

There are several ways in which and information system can be incorporated within an overall quality management plan:

- Case recording processes can be built around the MIS and its data entry forms.
- Reports can be generated to demonstrate performance at the staff and program level.
- Reports can be generated to determine if clients are receiving the specified program service components at the expected level.

OUTCOMES MEASURES

Outcomes are an important part of any quality management plan. Many home visitors are suspicious of the idea of measuring the results of their work (Clapp and Buake 1997; Carrilio et al. 2003). Outcomes are the results we expect if the services suggested by our program model are effective. It is important to recognize that the purpose of looking at outcomes is to identify what works and what does not. Sometimes home visitors feel this is a judgment of their work's quality. However, it is possible to do a very good job of something only to find that it cannot be shown to be effective in the sense of producing the expected results (Landsverk et al. 2001). Your job as a home visitor is to understand your program's services and model and to perform your work in a high quality manner. It is helpful if you are able to separate an evaluation of the program from an evaluation of *you*.

Often program administrators and funders decide the things that are to be measured. It is important for the home visitor to clearly understand how his/her activities with families relate to the expected program outcomes. A logic model, such as the one described in figure 2.3, is a good way to visualize the connection between the program goals, your activities, and the outcomes to be measured. It is a good idea to review your program's logic model regularly with your supervisor or your team so you can maintain a sense of how what you do on a daily basis with families is connected to the goals of the program.

QUALITY MANAGEMENT PLANS

A quality management plan outlines a process, which is intended to assure that programs operate according to standards of best practice. Quality programs carry out regular self-reviews to assure fidelity to standards and to provide a mechanism for introducing program improvements. A quality program will incorporate into its practice findings from self-studies, new information from the field and from current research. Home visitors are asked to document their work in order to help maintain program quality. A typical quality management plan might include

- Statement of the program concept and model
- Guidelines that define the components of the program and how they are expected to operate
- A self-evaluation tool, which indicates how well the program is meeting the guidelines

- Use of the self-evaluation tool at specified intervals
- A plan for responding to the findings of the self- evaluation

As part of your program's team you will be expected to participate in the quality management plan. The plan is usually the result of a great deal of preparation and discussion and represents the program's efforts to do the best job possible with families. The following description of what goes into the plan may help you to understand how your work fits in to the larger picture.

Statement of Program Concept and Model

The first step in managing quality is to identify what the program is. In order to do this, it is necessary to articulate the program's goals, target population, expected outcomes, service components, and standards of service. It is important to define how the program components are expected to work together.

Guidelines Defining Program Components

Based on the program concept, a detailed set of guidelines describing, in very concrete terms, the operational steps necessary to carry out the program needs to be developed. By assuring that the program is addressing each of the items listed in the guidelines, an initial step toward quality is made.

Self-Evaluation Tool

The program guidelines can be used to develop a self-study checklist. This checklist should also include quality criteria established by the program and all of its stakeholders. Essentially these criteria help the program to determine how well it is doing and should include a picture of what the ideal program would look like. The self-study affords the organization an opportunity to compare itself to the ideal and to identify ways in which it can move closer to that ideal. This checklist should be very specific and include items that identify the way in which, through documentation, the program is able to demonstrate its adherence to program principles.

Therefore the self-study checklist should be precise enough to identify such things as: 1) the expected time between intake and first service; 2) the time period in which assessments are expected to be completed; 3) the way in which data from the assessments is used in the individualized family service plan; and 4) the way in which the individualized family service plan is updated and reviewed. This self-study checklist should include looking at a randomly chosen set of case files.

Use the Self-Evaluation Tool

The self-study checklist the program develops should be applied at regular intervals. After the self-study checklist is complete, the process continues with a review of the findings. Many programs will want to seek assistance from an outside consultant or peer reviewer at this point in the process. These individuals serve as representatives of the ideal standards and help the program staff and administration to maintain this vision as they respond to the findings of the self-study checklist. It is important for all of the stakeholders, including client families, staff, administrators, and funders, to understand the results and to engage in a constructive, active problem-solving process to bring the program closer to the ideal that is set forth in the program guidelines and checklist.

Response Plan

As the results of the self-study process are reviewed, the program has an opportunity, with all of its key stakeholders, to identify constructive ways to move closer to the ideal. This process should result in a quality plan, which will spell out clearly the steps that will be taken to respond to the findings of the self-evaluation. The quality plan must be reviewed by key stakeholders at an agreed upon interval. Honest appraisals of progress will help the program and its stakeholders to determine the effectiveness of the responses to the self-study. However, even after the quality plan has been completed, the process of quality management and self-study continues. Ideally the program will reinstitute the self-study process at regular intervals. This enables the program to review policies and procedures, to update practices, and to introduce new learning.

SUMMARY

In this chapter the importance of evaluating practice is presented. Some of the reasons that home visitors are asked to document their work are explored. Outcomes and program effectiveness are introduced. The chapter explains specific elements of data collection. An example of how to write progress notes is provided. Home visitors and their supervisors are encouraged to attend to quality management and to develop strategies for managing quality. It is important that programs, like home visitors, reflect upon their activities and honestly evaluate their effectiveness in order to assure quality.

REFERENCES

Abidin, R. 1995. Parenting Stress Index. *Psychological Assessment Resources Inc.,* 16204 N. Florida Ave., Lutz, Florida, 33549.

ACE Study. Adverse Childhood Experiences Study. http://www.acestudy.org/aboutus.php (accessed March 3, 2006).

Ames, N. 1999. Social work recording: A new look at an old issue. *Journal of Social Work Education* 35 (2): 227–37.

Anda, R. F., C. L. Whitfield, V. J. Felitti, D. Chapman, V. J. Edwards, S. R. Dube, and D. F. Williamson. 2002. Alcohol-impaired parents and adverse childhood experiences: the risk of depression and alcoholism during adulthood. *Journal of Psychiatric Services* 53 (8): 1001–9.

Applegate, J., and J. M. Bonnovitz. 1995a. Winnicott's concepts of vulnerability and disturbance. In *The Facilitating Partnership.* Northvale, N.J.: Jason Aronson Inc. 59–80.

———. 1995b. Winnicott's developmental theory. In *The Facilitating Partnership.* Northvale, N.J.: Jason Aronson Inc. 27–58.

Bandura, A. 1994. Self-efficacy in Vilayanur S. Ramachaudran, ed., *Encyclopedia of Human Behavior.* Vol. 4. New York: Academic Press. 71–81.

Barlow, J., S. Stewart-Brown, H. Callaghan, J. Tucker, N. Brocklehurst, H. Davis, and C. Burns. 2003. Working in partnership: The development of a home visiting service for vulnerable families. *Child Abuse Review* 12 (3): 172–89.

Barrett, S. 1999. Information systems: An exploration of the factors influencing effective use. *Journal of Research on Computing in Education* 32 (1): 4–17.

Bavolek, S. J., and R. G. Keene. 1999. *Handbook for the AAPI-2: Adult-Adolescent Parenting Inventory.* Park City, Utah: Family Development Resources.

Bayley, N. 1993. *Bayley Scales of Infant Development.* 2nd ed. New York: Psychological Corporation.

Boyer, S. L., and G. R. Bond. 1999. Does assertive community treatment reduce burnout? A comparison with traditional case management. *Mental Health Services Research* 1 (1): 31–45.

Breakey, G. E., and B. Uohara-Pratt. 1991. Health growth for Hawaii's Healthy Start. *Zero to Three: Bulletin of the National Center for Clinical Infant Programs* 11 (4): 16–22.

Brilliant, E. L. 1986. Social work leadership—A missing ingredient. *Social Work.* 325–31.

Buchanan, A., F. Bennet, C. Ritchie, T. Smith, G. Smith, L. Harker, and S. Vitali-Ebers. 2004. The impact of government policy on social exclusion among children aged 0–13 and their families: A review of the literature for the social Exclusion Unit. In *Breaking the Cycle* series. London: Office of the Deputy Prime Minister. Social Exclusion Unit. http://www.socialexclusionunit.gov.uk/downloaddoc.asp?id=267 (accessed March 3, 2006).

Buka, S., and F. Earls. 1993. Early determinants of delinquency and violence. *Health Affairs* (Winter): 46–64.

Burke, A. C., and J. D. Clapp. 1997. Ideology and social work practice in substance abuse settings. *Social Work* 42 (6): 552–62.

Caldwell B., and R. Bradley. 1984. *Home Observation for Measurement of the Environment, (HOME).* rev. ed.. HOME INVENTORY LLC, Distribution Center, 2627 Winsor Drive, Eau Claire, WI 54703.

California State Senate. 1998. California Families and Children Home Visit Program. (S. B. 1525). http://www.sen.ca.gov/sor/reports/reports_by_year/1998/98issu17.htm (accessed May 13, 2005).

Carrilio, T. 1981. The impact of research in a family service agency. *Social Casework: The Journal of Contemporary Social Work* 62 (February 1981): 87–94.

———. 1998. The California Safe and Healthy Families Family Support (CAL-SAHF) home visiting model: Executive summary. California Office of Child Abuse Prevention. 2nd ed. San Diego, Calif.

———. 1999. *Curriculum Guidelines for ABC Center-based Services.* Technical paper presented to the California Department of Social Services Office of Child Abuse Prevention, Sacramento.

———. 2001. Family Support Program Development—Integrating Research, Practice and Policy. *Journal of Family Social Work* 6 (3): 53–78

———. 2003a. Learning from experience? A review of three California initiatives addressing the needs of vulnerable families. *Social Policy Journal* 2 (2/3): 5–25.

———. 2003b. *A Step by Step Guide to Home Visiting.* San Diego: San Diego State University Foundation.

———. 2005a. Management information systems: why are they underutilized in the social services? *Administration in Social Work* 29 (2): 43–61.

———. 2005b. Looking inside the "black box": a methodology for measuring program implementation and informing social services policy decisions. *Social Policy Journal* 4 (3/4): 1–17.

———. 2006. The elusive search for the silver bullet in prevention and family support programs for vulnerable families. *Social Work and Social Sciences Review* 12 (2): 5–28.

Carrilio, T. E., M. Adler, and B. Sheffield. 1999. *Management Information System Users Manual.* San Diego: Social Policy Institute.

Carrilio, T. E., T. R. Cohen, and A. Goldman. 1980. The team method of delivering services to the elderly: An interim report. *Journal of Jewish Communal Service* 52 (1): 56–62.

Carrilio, T., J. Kasser, and A. H. Moretto. 1985. Management information systems: Who is in charge? *Social Casework: The Journal of Contemporary Social Work* 66 (7): 417–23.

Carrilio, T., T. Packard, and J. D. Clapp. 2003. Nothing in—Nothing out: Barriers to the use of performance data in social service programs. *Administration in Social Work* 27 (4): 61–75.

Carrilio, T., T. Packard, L. Cannady, M. Darling, J. Chamberlin, L. Gamble, and T. Bergthold. 2002. *Final Report—Answers Benefiting Children Program Evaluation.* Technical report submitted to the California Department of Social Services Office of Child Abuse Prevention, San Diego.

Carrilio, T. E., and C. A. Walter. 1984. Mirroring and autonomy. *Child and Adolescent Social Work* 1 (3):143–52.

Carrilio, T., and Eisenberg, D. (1984). Preventing burnout through peer support. *Social Casework* 65 (5): 307–10.

Chaffin, M., B. L. Bonner, and R. F. Hill. 2001. Family preservation and family support programs: Child maltreatment outcomes across client risk levels and program types. *Child Abuse & Neglect* 25 (10): 1269–89.

Children's Hospital San Diego, Center for Child Abuse Prevention. 1994–1997. South Bay Home Support Project. Funded by the County of San Diego, San Diego, Calif.

Clapp, J. D., and A. C. Burke. 1997. Supervisor ideology and organizational response: HIV/AIDS prevention in outpatient substance abuse treatment units. *Administration in Social Work* 21 (1): 49–64.

———. 1999. Discriminant analysis of factors differentiating among substance abuse treatment units in their provision of HIV/AIDS harm reduction services. *Social Work Research* 23 (2): 69–76.

Clapp, J. D., A. C. Burke, and L. Stanger. 1998. The institutional environment, strategic response and program adaptation: A case study. *Journal of Applied Social Sciences* 22 (1): 87–95.

Clapp, J. D., and T. J. Early. 1999. A qualitative exploratory study of substance abuse prevention outcomes in a heterogeneous prevention system. *Journal of Drug Education* 29 (3): 217–33.

Congress, E .P. 1994. The use of culturagrams to assess and empower culturally diverse families. *Families in Society: The Journal of Contemporary Human Services* 75 (9): 531–38.

Copeland, V. C., and S. Wexler. 1995. Policy implementation in social welfare: A framework for analysis. *Journal of Sociology and Social Welfare* 22 (3): 51–68.

Cournoyer, B. 2004. *The Evidence-Based Social Work Skills Book.* New York: Allyn and Bacon.

Cowen, P. S. 2001. Effectiveness of a parent education intervention for at risk families. *Journal of the Society of Pediatric Nurses* 6 (2): 74–82.

Culross, P. L. 1999. Summary of home visiting program evaluation outcomes. *The Future of Children: Recent Program Evaluations* 9 (1): 195–223.

Daro, D. 2005. Letter to the editor: Response to Chaffin. *Child Abuse & Neglect* 29 (3): 237–40.

Daro, D., and A. C. Donnelly. 2002a. Charting the waves of prevention: Two steps forward, one step back. *Child Abuse & Neglect* 26 (6/7): 731–42.

Daro, D., and A. C. Cohn-Donnelly. 2002b. Child abuse prevention: Accomplishments and challenges. In *The A.P.S.A.C. Handbook on Child Maltreatment.* Edited by J. E. B. Meyers, L. Berliner, J. W. Briere, C. T Hendrix, C. Jenny, and T. Reid. Thousand Oaks, Calif.: Sage Publications. 431–48.

Daro, D., and K. Harding. 1999. Healthy Families America: Using research to enhance practice. *The Future of Children: Recent Program Evaluations* 9 (1): 152–76.

Daro, D., K. McCurdy, L. Falconnier, and D. Stojanovic. 2003. Sustaining new parents in home visitation services: Key participant and program factors. *Child Abuse & Neglect* 27 (10): 1101–25.

Davies, D. 1999. Risk and protective factors. In *Social Work Practice with Children and Families.* Edited by N. B. Webb. New York: Guilford Press. 44–83.

DeJong, P., and I. K. Berg. 2002. *Interviewing for Solutions.* 2nd ed. Pacific Grove, Calif: Brooks/Cole.

Domitrovich, C. E., and M. T. Greenberg. 2000. The study of implementation: Current findings from effective programs that prevent mental disorders in school-aged children. *Journal of Educational and Psychological Consultation* 11 (2): 93–221.

Donaldson, S. I., and M. Scriven. 2003. *Evaluating Social Programs and Problems.* Mahwah, N.J.: Lawrence Erlbaum Associates.

Dorsey, D. 2002. Information technology. In *Implementing Organizational Interventions.* Edited by J. Hedge and E. Pulkalos. San Francisco: Jossey-Bass. 110–32.

Dube, S. R, R. F. Anda, V. J. Felitti, D. P. Chapman, and W. H. Giles. 2003. Childhood abuse, neglect and household dysfunction and the risk of illicit drug use: The Adverse Childhood Experience Study. *Pediatrics* 111 (3): 564–72.

Duggan, A., E. McFarlane, A. Windham, C. Rohde, D. Salkever, L. Fuddy, L. Rosenberg, S. Buchbinder, and C. Sia. 1999. Evaluation of Hawaii's Healthy Start Program. *The Future of Children. Home Visiting: Recent Program Evaluations* 9 (1): 66–90.

Duggan, A., E. McFarlane, L. Fuddy, L. Burrell, S. M. Higman, A. Windham, and C. Sia. 2004. Randomized trial of a statewide home visiting program: Impact in preventing child abuse and neglect. *Child Abuse & Neglect* 28 (6): 597–622.

Eisenberg, D., and T. Carrilio. 1983. Informal resources for the elderly: Panacea or empty promise? *Journal of Gerontological Social Work* 6 (1): 39–47.

Emde, R. 1996. Developing a sense of self and others. *Zero to Three: Bulletin of the National Center for Clinical Infant Programs* 17 (1):17–24.

Erikson, E. 1963. The eight ages of man. In *Childhood and Society*. 2nd ed. New York: W. W. Norton. 247–74.

Erikson, M., and K. Kurz-Reimer. 1999. *Infants, Toddlers, and Families: A Framework for Support and Intervention*. New York: Guilford Press.

Everhart, K., and A. Wandersman. 2000. Applying comprehensive quality programming and empowerment evaluation to reduce implementation barriers. *Journal of Educational and Psychological Consultation* 11 (2): 177–91.

Ewing, J. 1984. Detecting alcoholism: The CAGE questionnarie. *Journal of the American Medical Association* 252 (14): 1905–07.

Family Support America. http://www.familysupportamerica.org/content/home.htm (accessed March 4, 2006).

Fitzgerald, B., and C. Murphy. 1994. Introducing executive information systems into organizations: Separating fact from fallacy. *Journal of Information Technology* 9 (4): 288–96.

Fitzpatrick, J. 2002. A conversation with Leonard Bickman. *American Journal of Evaluation* 23 (1): 69–80.

Fonagy, P. 1998. Prevention, the appropriate target of infant psychotherapy. *Infant Mental Health Journal* 19 (2): 124–50.

French, W., and C. Bell. 1998. *Organization Development: Behavioral Science Interventions for Organization Improvement*. 6th ed. Englewood Cliffs, N.J.: Prentice Hall.

The Future of Children. Home Visiting: Recent program evaluations 9 (1).

Gambrill, E. 2003. Evidence-based practice: Sea change or the emperor's new clothes? *Journal of Social Work Education* 39 (1): 3–23.

Garbarino, J. 1995. *Raising Children in a Socially Toxic Environment*. San Francisco: Jossey-Bass.

Garvin, D. A. 1993. Building a learning organization. *Harvard Business Review* 71 (4): 78–91.

Gavin, D. R., H. E. Ross, and H. A Skinner. 1989. Diagnostic validity of the drug abuse screening test in the assessment of DSM-III drug disorders. *British Journal of Addiction* 84 (3): 301–7.

Ghate, D., and M. Ramella. 2002. Positive parenting: The national evaluation of the youth justice board's parenting programme. London: Youth Justice Board for England and Wales, http://www.prb.org.uk/research%20projects/project%20summaries/p118.htm (accessed March 4, 2006).

Glisson, C. 2000. Organizational climate and culture. In *The Handbook of Social Welfare Management*. Edited by R. Patti. Thousand Oaks, Calif.: Sage Publications. 195–219.

Goetz, K., and S. Peck, eds. 1994. *The Basics of Family Support*. Chicago: Family Resource Coalition.

Gomby, D. 1999. Understanding evaluations of home visitation programs. *The Future of Children. Home Visiting: Recent Program Evaluations* 9 (1): 27–43.

Gomby, D., P. Culross, and R. Behrman. 1999. Home visiting: recent program evaluations—analysis and recommendations. *The Future of Children. Home Visiting: Recent Program Evaluation* 9 (1): 4–26.

Gomby, D., C. Larson, E. M. Lewitt, and R. Behrman. 1993. Home visiting: analysis and recommendations. *The Future of Children. Home Visiting* 3 (3): 6–22.

Guterman, N. B. 2001. *Stopping Child Maltreatment Before It Starts*. Thousand Oaks, Calif.: Sage Publications.

Hahn, R. A., J. Mercy, O. Bilukha, and P. Briss. 2005. Assessing home visiting programs to prevent child abuse: Taking silver and bronze along with gold. *Child Abuse & Neglect* 29 (3): 215–18.

Hall, J. A., C. Carswell, E. Walsh, D. L. Huber, and J. S. Jampoler. 2002. Iowa case management: Innovative social casework. *Social Work* 47 (2): 132–41.

Hancock, B. L., and L. Pelton.1989. Home visits: History and functions. *Social Casework* 70 (1): 21–27.

Harachi, T. W., R. D. Abbott, R. F. Catalano, K. P. Haggerty, and C. B. Fleming. 1999. Opening the black box: Using process evaluation measures to assess implementation and theory building. *American Journal of Community Psychology* 27 (5): 711–31.

Harvard Family Research Project (HFRP) http://www.gse.harvard.edu/hfrp/projects/ost_participation.html (accessed February 25, 2006).

Hasenfeld, Y., and R. Patti. 1992. The utilization of research in administrative practice. In *Research Utilization in the Social Services*. Edited by A. Grasso and I. Epstein. New York: Haworth Press. 221–39.

Healthy Families America. http://www.healthyfamiliesamerica.org/home/index.shtml (accessed February 27, 2006).

Heinicke, C., M. Goorsky, S. Moscov, K. Dudley, J. Gordon, C. Schneider, and D. Guthrie. 2000. Relationship-based intervention with at-risk mothers: Factors affecting variations in outcome. *Infant Mental Health Journal* 21 (3): 133–55.

Hepworth, D. H., R. H. Rooney, G. Dewberry Rooney, K. Strom-Gottfried, and J. A. Larsen. 2006. Countertransference reactions. In *Direct Social Work Practice: Theory and Skills*. 7th ed. Belmont, Calif.: Thomas Higher Education. 555–57.

Herie, M., and G. Martin. 2002. Knowledge diffusion in social work: A new approach to bridging the gap. *Social Work* 47 (1): 85–95.

Hernandez, M. 2000. Using logic models and program theory to build outcome accountability. *Education and Treatment of Children* 23 (1): 24–40.

Hodge, D. R. 2003. Differences in worldviews between social workers and people of faith. *Families in Society* 84 (2): 285–95.

Hodges, S., and M. Hernandez. 1999. How organizational culture influences outcome information utilization. *Evaluation and Program Planning* 22 (2): 183–97.

Hogue, A. 1996. Treatment adherence process research in family therapy: A rational and some practical guidelines. *Psychotherapy* 33 (2): 332–45.

Home Instruction Program for Parents of Preschool Youngsters (HIPPY). http://www.hippyusa .org/ (accessed February 26, 2006).

Horsch, K. 1996. Results-based accountability systems: Opportunities and challenges. *The Evaluation Exchange* 2 (1): 2–3.

Howe, D., M. Brandon, D. Hinings, and G. Schofield. 1999. *Attachment Theory, Child Maltreatment and Family Support: A Practice and Assessment Model.* Hampshire RG21 6XS: Macmillan Press.

Illig, D. 1998. *Birth to Kindergarten: The Importance of the Early Years.* California State Library. Monograph No. CR-98–001. Sacramento: California Research Bureau.

Jerrell, J., and M. S. Ridgely. 1999. The relative impact of treatment program robustness and dosage. *Evaluation and Program Planning* 22 (3): 323–30.

Johnson, D. W., and F. P. Johnson. 2006. Team development training in *Joining Together: Group Theory and Group Skills.* Boston: Allyn and Bacon, 530–65.

Julian, D., and J. D. Clapp. 2000. Planning, investment, and evaluation procedures to support coordination and outcomes based funding in a local United Way system. *Evaluation and Program Planning* 23 (1): 231–40.

Kagen, S. L., and P. Neville. 1993. *Integrating Services for Children and Families.* New Haven, Conn.: Yale University Press.

Kagen, S., D. Powell, P. Weisbourd, and E. Zigler, eds. 1987. *America's Family Support Programs.* New Haven, Conn.: Yale University Press.

Kagle, J. D. 1993. Record keeping: Directions for the 1990s. *Social Work* 38 (2): 190–96.

Karoly, L., P. Greenwood, S. Evringham, J. Hoube, M. R. Kilburn, P. Rydell, M. Saunders, and J. Chiesa. 1998. *Investing in Our Children: What We Know and Don't Know About the Costs and Benefits of Early Childhood Interventions.* Santa Monica: Rand Corporation.

Katz, I., and J. Pinkerton, eds. 2003. *Evaluating Family Support: Thinking Internationally, Thinking Critically.* Chichester, U.K.: John Wiley & Sons Ltd.

Kernberg, O. 1994. Aggression, trauma and hatred in the treatment of borderline patients. *Psychiatric Clinics of North America* 17 (4): 701–14.

Kettner, P. 2002. *Human Service Organizations.* Boston: Allyn and Bacon.

Kettner, P. M., R. Moroney, and L. Martin. 1999. Building a management information system. In *Designing and Managing Programs: An Effectiveness Based Approach.* 2nd ed. Thousand Oaks, Calif.: Sage Publications. 139–69.

Kitzman, H., D. L. Olds, C. R. Henderson Jr., C. Hanks, R. Cole, R. Tatelbaum, K. M. McConnochie, K. Sidora, D. W. Luckey, D. Shaver, K. Engelhardt, D. James, and K. Barnard. 1997. Effect of prenatal and infancy home visitation by nurses on pregnancy outcomes, childhood injuries, and repeated childbearing. A randomized controlled trial. *Journal of the American Medical Association* 278 (8): 644–52.

Klass, C. S. 1996. *Home Visiting: Promoting Healthy Parent and Child Development.* Baltimore: Paul H. Brookes Publishing Company Co.

Knitzer, J. 1999. *Promoting Resiliency Among the Most Stressed Young Children And Families: Toward More Responsive Welfare-Linked Policies and Programs.* National Center for Children in Poverty, Joseph L. Mailman School of Public Health, Columbia University. http://www .nccp.org/ (accessed March 1, 2006).

Kotter, J., and J. Heskett. 1992. *Corporate Culture and Performance*. New York: Free Press.

Kotulak, R. 1995. *Inside the Brain: Revolutionary Discoveries of How the Mind Works*. Kansas City: Andrews and McMeel.

Krugman, R. 1993. Universal home visiting: a recommendation from the U.S. Advisory Board on Child Abuse and Neglect. *The Future of Children: Home Visiting* 3 (3): 184–91.

Landsverk, J., T. E. Carrilio, C. Connelly, and W. Ganger. 2001. *Healthy Families San Diego: Final Technical Report*. Submitted to the California Department of Social Services, the Wellness Foundation, and Stuart Foundation. San Diego, Calif.: Child and Adolescent Services Research Center.

Lederer, A. L., and A. L. Mendelow. 1988. Convincing top management of the strategic potential of information systems. *MIS Quarterly* 12 (4): 525–34.

Leff, H. S., and V. Mulkern. 2002. Lessons learned about science and participation from multisite evaluations. In *New Directions for Evaluation*. Edited by J. M. Herrell and R. B. Straw. San Francisco: Jossey-Bass. 94: 89–100.

Lewandowski, C. A., and L. F. GlenMaye. 2002. Teams in child welfare settings: Interprofessional and collaborative processes. *Families in Society* 83 (3): 245–57.

Lewis, J., M. Lewis, T. Packard, and F. Souffle. 2001. Designing and using information systems. In *Management of Human Service Programs*. 3rd ed. Pacific Grove, Calif.: Brooks/Cole. 209–34.

Light, P. 2000. Making nonprofits work: a report on the tides of nonprofit management reform. Washington D.C.: Aspen Institute, Brookings Institution Press.

MacDonald, L., and T. V. Sayger. 1998. Impact of a family and school based prevention program on protective factors for high risk youth: Issues in evaluation. *Drugs and Society* 12 (1/2): 61–65.

MacMillan, H. L., B. H. Thomas, E. Jamieson, C. A. Walsh, M. H. Boyle, H. S. Shannon, and A. Gafni. 2005. Effectiveness of home visitation by public-health nurses in prevention of the recurrence of child physical abuse and neglect: a randomized controlled trial. *The Lancet* http://www.thelancet.com/ (accessed March 4, 2006).

Manolo, V., and W. Meezan. 2000. Toward building a typology for the evaluation of services in family support programs. *Child Welfare* 7 (4): 405–79.

Margie, N., and D. Phillips, eds. 1999. *Revisiting Home Visiting: A Summary of a Workshop*. Washington, D.C.: National Academy Press.

Mark, M. M. 2003. Toward an integrative view of the theory and practice of program and policy evaluation in S. I. Donaldson and M. Scriven, eds., *Evaluating Social Programs and Problems*. New Jersey: Lawrence Erlbaum Associates: 183–204.

Martin, J. B. 1999. Healthy families America. *The Future of Children. Home Visiting: Recent Program Evaluations* 9 (1): 177–78.

Martin, L. 2000. Performance contracting in the human services: An analysis of selected state practices. *Administration in Social Work* 24 (2): 29–44.

Marwell, N. P. 2004. Privatizing the welfare state: Nonprofit community-based organizations as political actors. *American Sociological Review* 69 (2): 265–91.

Maslow, A. 1954. *Motivation and Personality*. New York: Harper and Row.

Mayfield, D., G. McLeod, and P. Hall. 1974. The CAGE questionnaire: Validation of a new alcoholism screening instrument. *American Journal of Psychiatry* 13 (10): 1121–23.

McCurdy, K. 1995. *Home Visiting*. Chicago: National Committee to Prevent Child Abuse.

McCurdy, K., and D. Daro. 2001. Parent involvement in family support programs: An integrated theory. *Family Relations* 50 (2): 113–21.

McGuigan, W. M., A. R. Katzev, and C. Pratt. 2003. Multi-level determinants of retention in a home visiting child abuse prevention program. *Child Abuse & Neglect* 27 (40): 363–80.

McPhatter, A. R. 1991. Assessment revisited: a comprehensive approach to understanding family dynamics. *Families in Society: The Journal of Contemporary Human Services* 72 (1): 11–21.

Moore, S. T. 1998. Organizational and managerial supports for service quality in health and human services. *Family and Community Health* 21 (2): 20–30.

Mori Research Group. 2005. So called "hard to reach groups." Local Government Research Unit. www.mori.com/localgov/reach.php (accessed March 4, 2006).

Mrazek, P. J., and R. J. Haggerty, eds. 1994. *Reducing Risk for Mental Disorders: Frontiers for Preventive Intervention Research.* Washington, D.C.: National Academy Press, National Academy of Sciences.

Mutschler, E. 1992. Computers in agency settings. In *Research Utilization in the Social Services.* Edited by A. Grasso and I. Epstein. New York: Haworth Press. 325–44.

Mutschler, E., and Y. Hasenfeld. 1986. Integrated information systems for social work practice. *Social Work* 31 (5): 345–49.

National Center for Children in Poverty. http://www.nccp.org/ (accessed March 1, 2006).

Nunnally, J. 1967. *Psychometric Theory.* New York: McGraw-Hill.

O'Connor, G. G. 1988. Case management: System and practice. *Social Casework: The Journal of Contemporary Social Work* 69 (2): 97–106.

Ogborne, A. C., K Braun, and B. R. Rush. 1998. Developing an integrated information system for specialized addiction treatment agencies. *Journal of Behavioral Health Services and Research* 25 (1): 100–109.

Olds, D. L. 1999. The nurse home visitation program. *The Future of Children. Home Visiting: Recent Program Evaluations* 9 (1): 190–91.

———. 2003. Reducing program attrition in home visiting: What do we need to know? *Child Abuse & Neglect* 27 (4): 359–61.

Olds, D., and C. Henderson. 1989. The prevention of maltreatment. In *Child Maltreatment: Theory and Research on the Causes and Consequences of Child Abuse and Neglect.* Edited by D. Cichetti and V. Carlson. New York: Cambridge University Press. 722–63.

Olds, D. L., C. Henderson, H. Kitzman, J. Eckenrode, R. Cole, and R. Tattlebaum. 1999. Prenatal and infancy home visitation by nurses: Recent findings. *The Future of Children. Home Visiting: Recent Program Evaluations* 9 (1): 44–63.

Olds, D. L., and H. Kitzman. 1993. Review of research on home visiting for pregnant women and parents of young children. *The Future of Children: Home Visiting* 3 (3): 53–92.

Olds, D. L., H. Kitzman, R. Cole, J. Robinson, K. Sidora, D. W. Luckey, C. R. Henderson Jr., C. Hanks, J. Bondy, and J. Holmberg. 2004. Effects of nurse home visiting on maternal life course and child development: Age 6 follow-up results of a randomized trial. *Pediatrics* 114 (6): 1550–59.

Olds, D. L., J. Robinson, R. O'Brien, D. W. Luckey, L. M. Pettitt, R. K. Ng, K. L. Sheff, J. Korfmacher, S. Hiatt, A. Talmi, and C. R. Henderson Jr. 2002. Home visiting by paraprofessionals and by nurses: A randomized, controlled trial. *Pediatrics* 110 (3): 486–97.

O'Looney, J. 1997. Marking progress toward service integration: Learning to use evaluation to overcome barriers. *Administration in Social Work* 21 (3/4): 31–65.

Orwin, R. 2000. Assessing program fidelity in substance abuse health services research. *Addiction* 95 (supp. 13): S309.

Parents as Teachers. http://www.parentsasteachers.org/ (accessed March 3, 2006).

Pascoe, J. M., N. S. Ialongo, W. F. Horn, M. A. Reinhart, and D. Perrradatto. 1988. The reliability and validity of the Maternal Social Support Index. *Family Medicine* 20 (4): 271–76.

Patton, M. 1997. *Utilization-Focused Evaluation*. Thousand Oaks, Calif.: Sage Publications.

Pieper, M. 1994. Science, not scientism: The robustness of naturalistic clinical research. In *Qualitative Research in Social Work*. Edited by E. Sherman and W. Reid. New York: Columbia University Press. 71–88.

Pipp-Siegal, S., and L. Pressman. 1996. Developing a sense of self and others. *Zero to Three: Bulletin of the National Center for Clinical Infant Programs* 17 (1): 17–24.

Poertner, J. 2000. Managing for service outcomes. In *The Handbook of Social Welfare Management*. Edited by R. Patti. Thousand Oaks, Calif.: Sage Publications. 267–81.

Poole, D. L., J. Nelson, S. Carnahan, N. G. Chepenik, and C. Tubiak. 2000. Evaluating performance measurement systems in nonprofit agencies: The Program Accountability Quality Scale (PAQS). *American Journal of Evaluation* 21 (1): 15–26.

Prochaska, J. O., C. C. DiClemente, and J.C. Norcross. 1992. In search of how people change: Applications to addictive behaviors. *American Psychologist* 47 (9):1102–14.

Proctor, E. K. 2002.Quality of care and social work research. *Social Work Research* 26 (4): 195–97.

Proehl, R. 2001. *Organizational Change in the Human Services*. Thousand Oaks, Calif.: Sage Publications.

Radloff, L. S. 1977. The CES-D scale: A self-report depression scale for research in the general population. *Applied Psychological Measurement* 1: 385–401.

Rapp, C., and J. Poertner. 1992. *Social Administration: A Client-Centered Approach*. New York: Longman.

Rapp, C. A., and R. J. Goscha. 2004. The principles of effective case management of mental health services. *Psychiatric Rehabilitation Journal* 27 (4): 319–33.

Raudenbush, S. W., and A. S. Bryk. 2002. *Hierarchical Linear Models: Applications and Data Analysis Methods*. 2nd ed. Thousand Oaks, Calif.: Sage Publications.

Reynolds, A. J., J. Temple, D. Robertson, and E. Mann. 2001. Long term effects of an early childhood intervention on educational achievement and juvenile arrest: A 15-year follow-up of low-income children in public schools. *Journal of the American Medical Association* 285 (18): 2339–46.

Roberts-DeGennaro, M. 1993. Generalist model of case management. *Journal of Case Management* 2 (3): 106–11.

Rossi, P. H., H. Freeman, and M. Lipsey. 1999. *Evaluation: A Systematic Approach*. Thousand Oaks, Calif.: Sage Publications.

Royce, D., and B. Thyer. 1996. *Program Evaluation: An Introduction*. 2nd ed. Chicago: Nelson-Hall.

Rutter, M. Psychosocial resilience and protective mechanisms. *Journal of Orthopsychiatry* 57 (3): 316–31.

Saunders, J. B., O. G. Aasland, T. F. Babor, J. R. de la Fuente, and M. Grant. 1993. Development of the Alcohol Use Disorders Identification Test (AUDIT) WHO collaborative project on early detection of persons with harmful alcohol consumption. II. *Addiction* 88 (6): 791–804.

Schein, E. 1996. Leadership and organizational culture. In *The Leader of the Future*. Edited by F. Hesselbein, M. Goldsmith, and R. Beckhard. San Francisco: Jossey-Bass Inc. 59–69.

Scheirer, M. A. 2000. Getting more "bang" for your performance measures buck. *American Journal of Evaluation* 21 (2): 139–49.

Schoech, D. 1995. Information systems. In *Encyclopedia of Social Work*. 19th ed. Edited by R. Edwards. Washington, D.C.: NASW Press. 1470–79.

Schoech, D., D. Fitch, R. MacFadden, and L. Schkade. 2001. From data to intelligence: Introducing the intelligent organization. *Administration in Social Work* 26 (1): 1–21.

Schorr, L. 1997. *Common Purpose: Strengthening Families and Neighborhoods to Rebuild America*. New York: Doubleday.

Schorr, L., and D. Schorr. 1988. *Within Our Reach: Breaking the Cycle of Disadvantage*. New York: Doubleday.

Seligman, M. 1975. *Helplessness: On Depression, Development, and Death*. San Francisco: W. H. Freeman and Co.

Shera, W., and J. Page. 1995. Creating more effective human service organizations through strategies of empowerment. *Administration in Social Work* 19 (4): 1–15.

Sherwood, K. E. 2005. Evaluating home visitation: a case study of evaluation at the David and Lucile Packard Foundation. In *Teaching Evaluation Using the Case Method. New Directions for Evaluation*. No. 105. Edited by M. Q. Patton and P. Patrizi. San Francisco: Jossey-Bass. 59–78.

Shonkoff, J. P., and D. A. Phillips. 2000. *From Neurons To Neighborhoods: The Science of Early Childhood Development*. Washington, D.C.: National Academy Press.

———. 2001. From neurons to neighborhoods: The science of early childhood development—an introduction. *Zero to Three: Bulletin of the National Center for Clinical Infant Programs* 21 (5): 4–7.

Simmel, C. 2002. The Shared Family Care Development project: Challenges of implementing and evaluating a community based project. *Children and Youth Services Review* 24 (6–7): 455–70.

Sluyter, G. 1998. *Improving Organizational Performance*. Thousand Oaks, Calif.: Sage Publications.

Spotnitz, H. 1995. *Psychotherapy of Proedipal Conditions: Schizophrenia and Severe Character Disorders*. New York: Jason Aronson Publishers Inc.

Sprafkin, B. R. 1958. The meaning of the cost analysis study in the Jewish Family Service of Philadelphia. Presented at the Jewish Family Service Association of America Executive Conference. Chicago, Ill.

———. 1962. Gaining support for research and its use in a family agency: An administrator's responsibility. Presented at the National Conference on Social Welfare. Philadelphia, Pa.

Stein, L., and A. Santos. 1998. *Assertive Community Treatment of Persons with Severe Mental Illness*. New York: W. W. Norton and Co. Inc.

Stratham, J., and S. Holtermann. 2004. Families on the brink: the effectiveness of family support services. *Child and Family Social Work* 9 (2): 153–66.

Straus, M. A., S. L. Hamby, S. Boney-McCoy, and D. B. Sugarman. 1996. The Revised Conflict Tactics Scales (CTS2). *Journal of Family Issues* 17 (3): 283–316.

Straw, R. B., and J. M. Herrell. 2002. A framework for understanding and improving multisite evaluations. *New Directions for Evaluation* 94: 5–16.

Sweet, M. A., and M. I. Appelbaum. 2004. Is home visiting an effective strategy? A meta-analytic review of home visiting programs for families with young children. *Child Development* 75 (5): 1435–56.

Teague, G. 1998. Program fidelity in assertive community treatment: Development and use of a measure. *American Journal of Orthopsychiatry* 68 (2): 216–32.

Tichy, N. 1983. *Managing Strategic Change.* New York: John Wiley and Sons.

Tidmarsh, J., J. Carpenter, and J. Slade. 2003. Practitioners as gatekeepers and researchers: family support outcomes. *The International Journal of Sociology and Social Policy* 13 (1/2): 59–80.

U.S. Government Accounting Office. 1996. Effectively implementing the Government Performance and Results Act. http://www.gao.gov/special.pubs/gg96118.pdf (accessed March 4, 2006).

Van der Kolk, B., and R. Fisler. 1994. Childhood abuse and neglect and loss of self-regulation. *Bulletin of the Menninger Clinic* 58 (2): 145–68.

Van der Kolk, B., A. Hostetler, N. Herron, and R. Fisler. 1994. Trauma and the development of personality disorder. *Psychiatric Clinics of North America* 17 (4): 715–30.

Vinson, N. 2001. The system of care model: Implementation in 27 communities. *Journal of Emotional and Behavioral Disorders* 9 (1): 30–42.

Wagner, M., D. Spiker, M. I. Linn, S. Gerlach-Downie, and F. Hernandez. 2003. Dimensions of parental engagement in home visiting programs: Exploratory study. *Topics in Early Childhood Special Education* 23 (4): 171–87.

Walker, J. S., N. Koroloff, and K. Schutte. 2003. *Implementing High-Quality Collaborative Individualized Service/Support Planning: Necessary Conditions.* Portland, Ore.: Portland State University.

Walker, S. 2001. Family support and social work practice: Opportunities for child mental health work. *Social Work and Social Sciences Review* 9 (2): 25–40.

Walsh, J. 2003. *Endings in Clinical Practice: Effective Closure in Diverse Settings.* Chicago: Lyceum Books Inc.

Wasik, B. H., D. M. Bryant, J. J. Sparling, and C. T. Ramey. 1997. Maternal problem solving. In *Helping Low Birth Weight, Premature Babies: The Infant Health and Development Program.* Edited by R. T. Gross, D. Spiker, and C. Haynes. Palo Alto, Calif.: Stanford University Press. 276–89.

Webb. S. 2002. Evidence-based practice and decision analysis in social work: An implementation model. *Journal of Social Work* 2 (1): 45–63.

Weiss, H. 1993. Home visits: necessary but not sufficient. *The Future of Children. Home Visiting* 3 (3): 113–28.

Whyte, W., ed. 1991. *Participatory Action Research.* Newbury Park, Calif.: Sage Publications.

Winnicott, D. 1965. *The Maturational Processes and the Facilitating Environment.* New York: International Universities Press Inc.

Winter, M. M. 1999. Parents as teachers. *The Future of Children. Home Visiting: Recent Program Evaluations* 9 (1): 179–89.

Witkin, S. L., and W. D. Harrison. 2001. Whose evidence and for what purpose? *Social Work* 46 (4): 293–96.

Woods, P. A. 1999. Home instruction program for preschool youngsters (HIPPY). *The Future of Children. Home Visiting: Recent Program Evaluations* 9 (1): 192–94.

Woodside, M., and T. McClam. 2003. *Generalist Case Management: A Method of Human Service Delivery.* Pacific Grove, Calif.: Brookes/Cole-Thompson Learning.

Yin, R. K. 1993. *Applications of Case Study Research.* Thousand Oaks, Calif.: Sage Publications.

———. 1994. *Case Study Research: Design and Methods.* 2nd ed. Thousand Oaks, Calif.: Sage Publications

Yoshikawa, H. 1995. Long-term effects of early childhood programs on social outcomes and delinquency. *The Future of Children. Long Term Outcomes of Early Childhood Programs* 5 (3): 51–70.

Zeitz, M. A. 1995. The mothers' project: a clinical case management system. *Psychiatric Rehabilitation Journal* 19 (1): 55–62.

INDEX

abandonment, emotional, 101, 121, 124

acceptance, 6, 7, 36, 48, 50, 89

accountability, 26, 111

activities of daily living, 4, 15

administrative monitoring, 29, 36, 127–28, 133

administrative role in program design, 10, 110, 118

administrator attitudes and impact on programs, 21, 32–34, 38

administrators as stakeholders, 135

Adverse Childhood Experience (ACE) Study, 8

adverse consequences, 19

advocacy, advocates, 11, 19, 21

Aldrondo Family, 91

Amelia, 19

Assertive Case Management, 10, 15

assessment, 15, 52, 75–77, 94, 101, 134; of current functioning, 63; initial, 49; process, 56, 57; sample family assessment summary, 69; and service plan, 80–82; standardized tools, 68, 69; systematic, 39, 56–59, 76, 88, 99; write up, 69, 130

at risk, 6, 40

attachment, 4, 10, 18, 19, 24, 32, 41, 90, 110

authoritarian relationships, 47

autonomy, 1, 11, 14, 31, 33, 90, 121

baby steps, 81

barriers, 4, 43, 57, 63, 76, 77, 95, 102, 112, 113, 120

beginning, 23, 38, 39, 42, 44–47, 49, 59, 75, 81, 94, 100, 101, 103, 104, 107

Black Bear family, 92

boundaries, 31, 32, 40, 42, 48, 52, 91, 95, 113, 115, 122

brain research, 19, 90

Brown family, 131, 132

burnout, 111, 115

capacity, 1, 3, 15, 19, 37

carrying out the plan, 39, 56, 76, 88, 99

case management, 8, 10–15, 18, 20, 21, 26, 29, 34, 39, 40, 49, 56, 57, 59, 61, 67, 76, 99, 107, 110–3, 118, 119, 127, 132; case-management function, 12, 13, 34, 112; case-management process, 39, 49, 56, 67, 76, 88, 99; family-support case management, 39, 57, 59, 61, 67, 107; home-visiting case management, 49, 56, 76, 118; individual case management, 13; shared case management, 111. *See also* integrated-team case management; team case management

case record, 128–30, 132

case termination summary, 107, 108

caseload size, 29

center-based groups, 15, 119, 123

center-based services, 11, 15, 123

change, 11, 16, 17, 48, 63, 67, 75, 107; motivation to change, 51, 57, 67; process of change, 67, 68, 75, 103; readiness to change, 51, 59, 67, 68, 69; stages of change, 68, 75; theory of change, 40

"change is hard," 67

child abuse, 4, 10, 22, 40, 48, 59, 68

child development, 3, 17, 18, 25–27, 29, 32, 41, 48, 53, 54, 74, 92, 93, 96, 97, 108, 110, 119, 120, 127. *See also* development

cognitive development, 3, 10, 18, 19, 108. *See also* development

collaboration, 36, 41

communication, 36, 50, 51, 114

community context, 20, 57, 91, 118

community resources, 4–6, 12, 13, 15, 110

computers, 144

confidentiality, 48, 49, 129, 130

consistency, 11, 22, 31, 42, 113, 114, 122, 123, 128

continuity, 1, 11, 18, 36, 42, 43, 46, 59, 91, 95, 96, 101, 111, 114